Kinetic Awareness

DISCOVERING YOUR BODYMIND

Ellen Saltonstall

Kinetic Awareness Center

Library of Congress Cataloging-in-Publication Data

Saltonstall, Ellen.
Kinetic awareness.

Bibliography: page 75.
1. Mind and body therapies. I. Title.
RC489.M53S35 1988 615.8'51 88-1216
ISBN 0-89062-232-9

Designed by Romeo Enriquez.

Ornamental artwork is from William Rowe's *Original Art Deco Designs* published by Dover Publications, Inc. in 1973.

Photograph credits: Sophie Ludwig, 20; Philip Hipwell, 26; Tom Haynes, 32, 42, 44, 46, 51, 53; Amy Guggenheim, 48, 50.

Produced by the Publishing Center for Cultural Resources, New York City. Manufactured in the United States of America.

Contents

Acknowledgments

My thanks go first to Elaine Summers, without whom my life undoubtedly would have taken a very different course. She has been not only an enormously influential teacher and mentor for my professional development but a true friend through many years.

Michelle Berne, a colleague and friend, provided the initial inspiration to begin this project and has been extremely helpful and supportive. I thank her and my other colleagues in Kinetic Awareness—Robin Powell, Nannette Sievert, and Alexandra Ogsbury—for our discussions and shared experiences, which have helped immeasurably to form my understanding of the work.

Thanks also to my family for their patience and support in the process of producing this book, and to my students for the opportunity to make the work come alive for others as it has for me.

I am very grateful to my editor, Mary Kathryn Stillwell, whose enthusiasm and skills not only offered a fresh perspective but gave the project momentum. Thanks to photographers Tom Haynes and Amy Guggenheim, and to the students who modeled—Marie Casey, Arlene Greenberg, John Milich, and Caroline Simonds—for their help in illustrating the text. Special thanks to Sophie Ludwig for allowing me to print her photograph of Elsa Gindler.

M. J. Gladstone and the staff at the Publishing Center for Cultural Resources have facilitated the production process with expertise and graciousness. Others whose interest and support for the project have been helpful are Jean Balderston, Irene Dowd, Judith Katz, Joyce Morgenroth, and Wendy Rogers.

The practice of Siddha Yoga has had a profound effect on my life at many levels, both professional and personal. My spiritual teacher, Gurumayi Chidvilasananda, has sustained and supported me through her teachings and her love, and for this I thank her with all my heart.

Preface

I moved to New York City in 1971 to study dance. This followed years of training, first as an undergraduate at Cornell University, then at the University of California at Berkeley, where I had gone to do graduate work in education. My days in New York were busy ones, filled with technique classes and hours of rehearsal.

In many ways, I was a typical young dancer with plenty of enthusiasm and energy. I was also typical in that I had no knowledge of how to care for my body as an instrument. Before long, I developed a chronic knee problem. Fortunately, I was referred to several bodywork practitioners, among them Elaine Summers. I remember sitting and talking with her about her work during the spring of 1972. I was impressed by her assumption that anyone who chose to could become totally aware of and articulate with every part of the body. This was indeed an inspiring thought for a dancer.

What started as a way of recovering from my knee problem soon became a way of life. Although initially skeptical of the subtlety and gentleness of Kinetic Awareness, I appreciated its fundamental premise of going directly to the body for healing from the beginning. Soon, however, I became addicted to the pleasures of the work itself.

Today, awareness training is a part of the curriculum in many prominent college dance departments in the United States, but in 1972, it was definitely out of fashion. My dance colleagues were politely tolerant, but clearly, and almost exclusively, interested in traditional modern dance technique classes. I persisted, continuing with both kinds of study—the inward and the outward—at the same time.

For five years, I took weekly private classes in Kinetic Awareness with Nannette Sievert, who had been trained by Summers. During that time I also took whatever group classes Summers herself offered, and from 1973–75 I was a member of Summers' dance company, performing in her choreography, which was based on Kinetic Awareness skills and principles. Kinetic Awareness soon became a foundation of my development as a dancer, and, as I would realize later, as a teacher, as a parent, as a human being.

After this first period of intensive study, I began to teach Kinetic Awareness on a limited basis. Dancer friends who observed me doing awareness work and saw its benefits were eager to learn more. I also had trained in muscular therapy with Ben Benjamin, obtained a license to practice therapeutic massage, and established a private practice composed primarily of other dancers. Many of those who came to me for massage needed something that they could do for themselves, and gradually I introduced Kinetic Awareness to them.

I soon became aware that dancers are not the only ones who suffer from injuries and all sorts of chronic aches and pains. People of all types, professions, ages, sizes, and shapes need ways to improve their body useage, to become comfortable in their bodies, and to avoid both physical and psychological stress. While Kinetic Awareness was not widely known among dancers, however, it was even less well known to the general public.

During this time, I also undertook an ongoing study of Siddha Yoga, a spiritual practice of meditation originating in India. It was brought to the West by Swami Muktananda in the early 1970s and is currently taught by his successor, Swami Chidvilasananda. Kinetic Awareness and meditation have much in common, as I will discuss in Chapter 5. Briefly, both recognize the value of turning inside, finding resources deeper than our normal daily consciousness. Working with my body became part of a meditative process. Later, when I began to teach Hatha Yoga, the branch of yoga comprised of physical exercises, my background in therapeutic bodywork found yet another application.

In 1978, I began to study Kinetic Awareness more deeply from a theoretical point of view and to train more seriously as a teacher. In the process, I learned about the origins of Kinetic Awareness in Europe during the early part of this century and Summers' subsequent development of it in the United States since the 1960s. In order to put Kinetic Awareness in a perspective with that history, I enrolled in a master's degree program at New York University's Gallatin Division, where I studied biomechanics, kinesiology, other body therapies, and related subjects. The research lead to a thesis on Kinetic Awareness that is the basis of this book.

As part of my research, I interviewed a number of men and women who, like myself, have benefited from Kinetic Awareness. Some had come to it as I had, to recover from injuries. Others came for personal growth or for the sheer pleasure it gave them. Some were older, others young. A taxi driver and polo player, a singer and composer, an opera director, a nurse, several dancers, performance artists, and others recounted their experiences with Kinetic Awareness and the part it has played in their lives.

Since I received my degree in 1983, I have been fortunate to maintain my close association with Elaine Summers. She has in recent years established a teacher training program, and I am among several whom she has certified to teach Kinetic Awareness and to train other teachers.

My impetus to write this book came from a desire to bring the full scope of Kinetic Awareness theory and practice to the attention of a wider public, to those who are curious and who might benefit from this gentle, potent discipline. I hope this familiarity with Kinetic Awareness will inspire you to try it for yourself.

1

Kinetic Awareness as a Holistic Therapy

Throughout the twentieth century, investigators from a variety of fields have followed remarkably parallel and often overlapping paths exploring human nature. While psychologists and physicians have determined how mental stress can cause real physical ailments, educators have noted that a relaxation of the body can bring about a calm mind. Through their discoveries, the various aspects of our functioning come together to form an integrated picture of human nature, one in which the whole is more than the sum of its parts.

During this time, we have also opened ourselves to views that differ radically from the conventional Western perspective. The Chinese system of acupuncture meridians and the Yogic system of chakras, for example, have expanded our understanding of health as well as of sickness. Men and women from virtually every walk of life have reached out in many directions, varying from the age-old spiritual and physical disciplines such as meditation, Yoga, and T'ai Chi Ch'uan to newer ways such as experimentation with mind-altering drugs.

What has emerged from these many avenues of exploration has been a new, holistic approach to the therapeutic process, one that acknowledges the subtleties of human functioning. The aim of this approach—called "holistic" because it involves both mind and body—is to achieve more significant and lasting results than either mental or physical therapy could achieve separately. There is a strong "self-help" component in the approach and in the therapies that have grown from it.[1] This self-help aspect fills the gap between medical care and education and in this way fits into the pattern of the "human potential movement," which emphasizes personal growth and understanding.

As we increasingly realize that our thoughts and behavior influence our health and that our health affects our emotional and intellectual selves, the concept of "bodymind," or unity of our overall experiences, emerges. The traditional wisdom that the body "feels" and the mind "thinks"—and that experts are needed to mediate between the two—is now seen as too simplistic. Our own experience tells us that the mind and body must be approached together in order to answer a wide variety of important questions that arise in our daily lives. For example, why do certain moods give us tremendous physical energy, while others make us lethargic? Why are some strenuous activities tiring to some people and invigorating to others? What are our postural preferences, that is, the ways we tend to use our bodies in daily life, and how do they affect our sense of well-being? How is our emotional state reflected in our physical appearance and our ways of using our body?

While all of these questions, and many others, need to be addressed by any holistic method, such a method must have a starting point from which to work. Many start by examining mental attitudes, assuming that as the mind gradually releases tensions, corresponding tensions will be released in the body. Others, often called the "body therapies," examine the body's appearance, posture, tension patterns, movements, and habits, and note corresponding effects on the mind and emotions. A person whose body mechanics (the workings of the muscles and joints) are inefficient will experience unnecessary pain and fatigue. Efficient use, on the other hand, is rewarded by feelings of calm, strength, endurance, and flexibility. Improved musculoskeletal functioning, achieved with the involvement of the conscious mind, results in positive effects in the mental and emotional spheres, an enjoyment of the fully integrated self. In other words, when we are not working against ourselves, we have more energy and feel better.

The particular body therapy that I will discuss in the following pages is Kinetic Awareness. Although it shares theoretical and methodological bases with other bodymind systems, it is unique in many ways. My own experience and that of my students, as well as my research, have made it clear to me that its unique aspects make it particularly appropriate for a variety of people. Those who are suffering from specific problems—stress, muscle pain and stiffness, insomnia, chronic fatigue, or depression, for example—can benefit. And so can those who wish to learn from and about their bodies so that they can enjoy a richer, more comfortable life.

The benefits of Kinetic Awareness

As I prepared for my thesis and began interviewing students, I not only saw how diverse their backgrounds were but also discovered just how far-reaching the rewards of Kinetic Awareness work were. I have included some of their comments throughout the book to provide a wider perspective of the work and of the benefits you might expect. Here are five of the men and women whose experiences you will encounter in the pages that follow:[2]

Sue Shapiro, a clinical psychologist and psychoanalyst, came to Kinetic Awareness when she had just started doing Yoga and developed lower back pain. She continued her work because of the personal satisfaction it gave her even after her problems with poor leg alignment were resolved. "It's private and it's very much your own experience . . . it gets you in touch with your own resources," she says.

Tom Ollendorff, a polo player and cab driver, suffers from chronic migraines and asthma. When he began the work, he was bothered by stooped posture and an overall feeling of tension. He found that he could intervene in the tension patterns of an asthma or migraine attack using Kinetic Awareness techniques and in so doing often reduce his need for medication.

Fenna Koppelman, a public health nurse, suffered from headaches and from discomfort in one hip. She had been to several different medical specialists but was not satisfied by their treatment. Through Kinetic Awareness, which Fenna describes as a "common-sense approach," she learned how to adjust her posture and daily activities to avoid physical strain and how to relieve unnecessary tension. She sees a wide range of benefits for children as well as adults.

Linda Montano, a video and performance artist, did not come to Kinetic Awareness as a result of an ailment, but saw it as an ongoing part of her personal and artistic development.

Tony Nunziata, an actor and singer, made use of Kinetic Awareness as a technique to take care of his body and to enhance his expressive range. He says the work is an "everyday living and working tool," one that is experiential rather than intellectual. He appreciates that in Kinetic Awareness "you learn to internalize an awareness, an understanding of everything about the inside of your body."

These are only a few examples; Kinetic Awareness has helped many people find answers to physical problems and symptoms of stress. As well as relieving immediate symptoms, it can offer the student a fuller sense of the bodymind as a "total instrument for living," as it was described by an early pioneer of awareness work, Elsa Gindler.[3] I often think of it as a way to become a witness to your own being, and in that way it has much to offer healthy, happy people in terms of personal growth. The key concept is awareness itself.

The word "awareness" is usually used in a social sense: being aware of other people's feelings, of communication styles, group dynamics, or psycho-social-political trends. Other similar words are "consciousness," which implies an inward, more sophisticated awareness, and "sensitivity," which implies an awareness of things outside the body, perceived through the senses. As used by Elaine Summers, the word "awareness" really includes both "consciousness" and "sensitivity"; it is the state or activity of listening to messages from one's physical and emotional selves and observing one's outward behavior and environment.

The kinesthetic sense

Since Western culture's view of the physical body emphasizes how we look and how we hurt, it should be no surprise that our conventional education includes extensive training for the five senses of hearing, sight, taste, touch, and smell but ignores the "sixth" sense. This kinesthetic or proprioceptive sense tells us the positions of our body parts: the range, force, and timing of our movements; the tension in our muscles; our breathing pattern; our weight; and our overall sense of body image. It is usually only brought into play when investigating pain or disease, as if we should be aware only of discomforts and not of healthy functioning.

Perhaps our education has taught us that what we see and what we hear in the outside world are the most important perceptions to assimilate, so that we've developed them to the exclusion of others. Perhaps we feel that paying attention to ourselves inwardly in this way is self-centered or unnecessary because our body will function by itself until it sends out clear signals for help. All of these notions serve to suppress our kinesthetic sense and rob us of this great inner resource.

Kinetic Awareness is based on the premise that refinement of the kinesthetic sense, especially with regard to movement (hence the name "kinetic"), can bring about the gradual reintegration of bodymind functioning. The goal is not only to notice and be able to change situations that cause us pain but also to enjoy our daily selves when we are well. It is in this sense that Kinetic Awareness is much more than a therapy.

But what is Kinetic Awareness really like? What happens in class? Are there special techniques for special problems? How is it unique in the field of holistic body-oriented techniques? Can I work on my own? In what ways can it help me? How can I find a certified teacher? I hope to answer these and many other questions about the process and benefits of Kinetic Awareness in the pages that follow. First, however, I would like to tell you something about the various ideas and the climate of the times that lead to its birth during the early part of our century and of its subsequent development in both Europe and the United States.

Notes

1. The word "therapy" is perhaps inaccurate to describe the holistic systems I will be discussing, but as a working term appropriate to the systems, it denotes relief from discomfort and the restoration of good health.

2. Most of the men and women quoted in this book were interviewed in New York during 1981–82. Their contribution to my understanding of Kinetic Awareness has been invaluable, and I thank them for their cooperation. In most cases I have used their actual names.

3. "*Gymnastik* for Busy People," *Bulletin: Elsa Gindler 1885–1961*, vol. I, no. 10 (Caldwell, N.J.: Charlotte Selver Foundation, Summer 1978): page 37 (originally published in German in 1926 in the journal of the *Deutscher Gymnastik-Bund* [German *Gymnastik* Federation]).

2

The History of Kinetic Awareness

Elaine Summers came to awareness work as a dancer.[1] Trained in ballet as a child, Summers had continued to study dance while she majored in art education at the Massachusetts College of Art. After graduation, she worked as an art teacher and then a dance teacher before moving to New York in 1952 to study dance at the Juilliard School.

Summers studied independently with a number of prominent teachers,[2] and in the early 1960s she became a part of the innovative Judson Dance Theatre, a group of young experimental choreographers. In her performance work, she began to explore ways of incorporating not only the modern dance vocabulary but also ordinary movement, film, and music into a resulting "intermedia."

Throughout her training, Summers experienced the usual collection of dancer's injuries. As she sought medical treatment and advice on injury prevention, she soon realized that the medical profession had too narrow a view of possible treatments for injuries to the muscles and ligaments so often suffered by dancers. She also discovered that most dancers knew very little about how their bodies actually worked and even less about how to take care of them.

Summers' study at Juilliard was interrupted at 28 when she began to show symptoms of osteoarthritis, a potentially crippling disease of the joints, and it was at that time that her attention turned toward awareness work. The actual impetus came from a dream she had, in which she saw the possibility of doing dance movements easily, without strain. She related the dream to a therapist friend, Renee Nell, who referred her to Charlotte Selver and Carola Speads, former students of Elsa Gindler in Germany.

Summers studied with Selver for one year, then began a long association with Carola Speads in 1955. Studying in particular the writings of Wilhelm Reich, Summers also began to investigate the bodymind connection from the psychological as well as physical point of view.

These influences from earlier practitioners of healing arts, combined with Summers' own needs to deal with her body, led to the development of her own system of therapeutic work during the next fifteen years. Kinetic Awareness would provide relief not only to Summers and other ailing dancers but to countless others suffering from a variety of complaints. It would also provide a means whereby anyone who chose to undertake the exploration could enjoy the process of reawakening the bodymind.

The psychological perspective

To Freud, the founder of psychoanalysis, the mind and the body were intimately connected. Conflict within the personality, he discovered, could result in both mental and physical symptoms. He observed that physical symptoms, such as paralysis or numbness, could be brought about by the unconscious repression of ungratified desires or deep-seated fears. His method of treatment was to stimulate a release of memories, feelings, and associations so that repressed feelings could be expressed and physical symptoms relieved. While he did not treat the body directly, his work led other researchers to examine the bodymind connections more closely.

Wilhelm Reich, a student of medical and psychoanalytic sciences in Vienna in the 1920s, worked as a young psychoanalyst in Freud's clinic.[3] There he was able to examine Freud's theories and methods firsthand. Although the whole scope of Reich's work is even more controversial than Freud's, his contributions to the understanding of bodymind interaction are reflected in the underlying assumptions of many recent bodymind techniques such as Rolfing and Bioenergetics.

Briefly, Freud and Reich both agreed that blocked sexual energy—such as in patients with severe sexual inhibitions—behaved like a toxic substance in the body. It caused purely somatic symptoms such as backaches and headaches. Freud distinguished between patients whose neuroses were somatically linked and those whose were purely psychic, although sexually, related. Reich, on the other hand, felt that there could never be such a separation between mind and body. He saw, for example, the orgasm as a functional necessity for a person's total health, maintaining that the cycle of excitation through release is necessary for both mental and physical well-being.

As Reich treated patients, letting them talk without his interaction, he noticed that most of them had resistances to the therapeutic process, which were experienced both verbally and physically. He called this resistance "character armor." The way in which things were said or not said (in a patient's bodily behavior), he believed, told as much as the actual verbal material. In working more directly with "character resistances," or the particular ways in which people protected themselves, he developed his technique of Character Analysis.

Here Reich diverged radically from Freud's technique by saying that the sequence of the treatment was not fixed. The analyst did not have to deal with associations from a patient's childhood right away because a large part of the psychological problem was usually the resistance to the therapy itself, and Reich found he could deal with this directly.

Character armor proved to be the link to discovering how directly the body is involved in mental functioning. Reich found that these resistances always expressed themselves in the body. Again breaking the rules of Freudian analysis by touching his patients, he realized that he could work on the physical resistances directly. Releasing the physical energies brought a flood of psychological material out of hiding. Reich described his findings:

> In a short time I had a profusion of facts at my disposal. They reduced themselves to concise formulation: sexual life energy can be bound by chronic muscular tensions. Anger and anxiety can also be blocked by muscular tensions. From now on, I found that whenever I dissolved a muscular tension, one of the three basic biological excitations of the body, anxiety, hate, or sexual excitation, broke through. I had, of course, succeeded in doing this before through the loosening of purely characterological inhibitions and attitudes. But now the breakthroughs of vegetative energy were more complete, more forceful, experienced more affectively and occurred more rapidly. In the process, the characterological inhibitions were loosened spontaneously. . . . Quite rapidly, a number of decisive questions pertaining to the relationship between mind and body were clarified. . . . Muscular attitudes and character attitudes have the same function in the psychic mechanism. They can replace one another and be influenced by one another. Basically, they cannot be separated. They are identical in their function.[4]

Reich began to look more closely at the body as an indicator of a patient's mental state and to observe how the muscular tensions, or body armor, functioned and how it reacted to treatment. He saw that whenever there was internal energy that could not be discharged because of inhibitions, armor would form in the muscles and prevent further c energy. He observed, for example, that "inhibited pleasure is t into rage, and inhibited rage is transformed into muscular spasms."

He noted that the body language is not always translatable, however, and a great variation exists in the types of expressions that are contained in various types of body armor. Therapies that developed later—and owe a great debt to Reich's discoveries—are often too quick to make standardized connections. Suppressed anger, for example, is said to cause upper back tension, or suppressed sadness is said to cause jaw tension. Reich, on the other hand, acknowledged the responsibility of the therapist to remain open to exactly what was being expressed by each individual patient. His only generalization in this regard was to say that when armor existed, something was being held back:

> The total expression of the armored organism is one of restraint. The meaning of this expression is quite literal: the body is expressing that it is holding back. Pulled-back shoulders, thrust-out chest, rigid chin, superficial, suppressed breathing, hollowed-out loins, retracted, immobile pelvis . . . are the essential attitudes and mechanisms for total restraint.[6]

A difficult situation in a patient's childhood would become pathological later only if associated body armor developed and persisted over long periods of time. Such an armor could, however, be released by moving the affected part of the body in certain ways to encourage the tension to release mechanically, or by manipulations by the therapist. Sometimes new armor would form, he found, as a reaction to the release of tension, since the armor functioned as a defense. Reich's therapeutic method aimed at opening up the patient's means of expression, both in body language and in verbal language, so that energy that naturally flowed out of a person could do so without blocks.

Elsa Gindler

Reich developed his theories about bodymind connections in the 1920s and '30s, a time of great political upheaval. After working in Vienna and Berlin, he had been forced to leave Europe and to complete his work in Norway and the United States. At the same time, a woman in Berlin named Elsa Gindler was teaching what she called *Arbeit am Menschen*, "work on the human being."[7] Gindler's work came out of a physical-education context rather than psychoanalysis, but the shared foundations are astonishing and are fundamental to the body therapies that developed

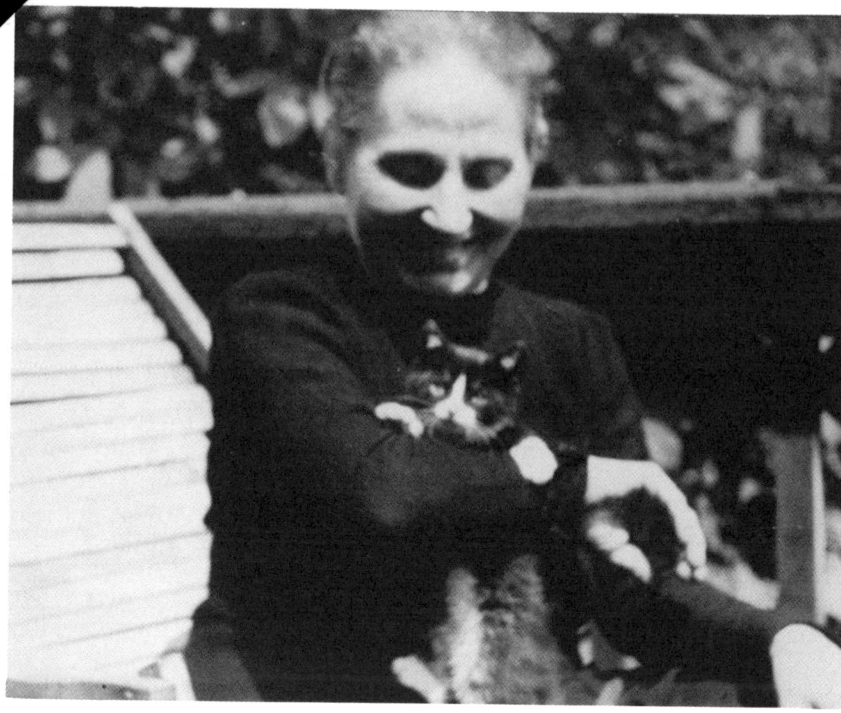

Elsa Gindler in 1946.

later. Both Reich and Gindler worked with the understanding that the psyche structures the body to satisfy its needs and that therapeutic bodywork can affect both the body and the emotions.

In Germany in the early 1920s, the prevailing system of physical education was pre-military training for boys and men, emphasizing muscle-building, calisthenics, and competitive sports. In response to that, several women introduced a different approach for girls and women, which they called *Gymnastik*, the purpose of which was to foster development of natural movement, coordination, rhythm, and the emotional expression of the individual. The two main proponents of *Gymnastik* were Hede Kallmeyer and Bess Mensendieck, both of whom had studied with Genevieve Stebbins in America.[8]

Although *Gymnastik* was separate from the public school system in Germany, it became an established (though still revolutionary) professional teaching field, regulated by the government and requiring three years of training. Gindler studied with Kallmeyer, whose goal it was to revise the standard physical education for children in Germany so that it encouraged freedom of movement rather than "exercise." As a young teacher, Gindler was already interested in the challenge of keeping the body healthy and strong without sacrificing a sensitivity and curiosity about exploring our natural physical capacities. She became a central figure in the *Gymnastik* movement, acting as president of the German Association of *Gymnastik* teachers.

As often happens with innovators, Gindler developed her subsequent original work in response to her own needs. In her twenties she was diagnosed with incurable tuberculosis. Instead of the retreat to the pure mountain air that her doctors recommended, she believed that if she could become extremely sensitive to her own processes, she could aid the body's natural healing powers. She concentrated on the breathing process so carefully and with such patience and persistence that she was able to rest the diseased lung and breathe mostly with the healthy lung, a skill which would seem impossible to most people. In a year she was cured, and what she had learned became the basis of the rest of her life's work.

In "*Gymnastik* for Busy People," Gindler cuts through the complexities of the psychoanalytical approach to the bodymind unity as she defines her work:

> It is difficult for me to speak about *Gymnastik* because the aim of my work is not learning certain movements, but rather the achievement of concentration. Only by means of concentration can we attain the full functioning of the physical apparatus in relation to mental and spiritual life. We therefore advise our students from the very first lesson that our work must be pursued consciously: it can only be entered into and understood through consciousness. . . . By that I mean consciousness that is centered, reacts to the environment and can think and feel. I deliberately avoid defining this consciousness as soul, psyche, mind, feeling, subconsciousness, individuality, or even the 'body-soul.' For me the small word 'I' summarizes all this. . . . It is clear that merely learning and doing these *Gymnastik* exercises cannot lead to the attainment of full consciousness. How do we get closer to that? Simply by using all our spirit and feeling in bringing our body to be a responsive instrument for living.[9]

At the outset, Gindler's students were encouraged to become attuned to everything that happened in their bodies, then to let go of what was not needed for full, healthy functioning. Changes would come from within the body, not from an external idea of what the body should look like or how a person should breathe. She began to call the activities in the class "experiments" rather than "exercises," so that students would do them with a sense of discovery and nonjudgmental openness toward what might happen or what they might feel.

Gindler felt that there was a natural and unique quality to the way each person's body functioned, which should be respected and nurtured. By working in a concentrated way to experience what was actually happening in the body, one could best cooperate with the body's innate drive toward full, healthy functioning. Her classes dealt with the particular body problems that her students complained of but also focused on four general, interrelated topics: breathing, relaxation, tension, and gravity.

Breathing, she said, is subtly connected with all the movements that we make, and the constriction of one impedes the other. Difficult situations in our lives cause us to cramp our breathing, which reduces our possibilities of reacting with full mental or physical capacity. Her students would often work for weeks on simply letting the breathing go on without interfering with it. "Constricted breathing," she wrote, "is closely related to unhealthy physical tension: we can never reach physical ease if the activity of breathing is not simultaneously freed of all constriction."[10]

Relaxation of unwanted tension in the body was an ongoing concern, and she made it clear just what kind of relaxation she meant; it wasn't collapsed inertia.

> For us relaxation is that condition in which we have the greatest capacity of reacting. It is a stillness within us, a readiness to respond appropriately to any stimulus. This is the kind of relaxation we are seeking. It can be most readily reached through the experience of gravity.[11]

Gravity must be experienced and understood throughout all the limbs of the body: how the feet give the weight to the ground, how the spine feels when standing or sitting, and how the head rests when lying down. When we feel the weight of the body, Gindler pointed out, "nature takes over the work for us," and we are more available for free movements and easy breathing.[12]

As students set out to work therapeutically on particular problems in their bodies, they would start by just sensing what was happening inside and letting the body indicate what changes might bring about improvements, such as less pain or more ease in movement. Changes were gradual, and there were always accompanying mental changes. Gindler's student Charlotte Selver writes:

> We found that such changes are closely related to changes in our attitudes; in fact we found out that they are the same. When a person changed in his "physical" balance, he also became more balanced as a person. When someone was able to give up his "physical" overdoings he became more peaceful and open as a person. In other words, there was nothing that

> would not work in both directions at once within oneself. Gin more and more interested in that, and by and by she bega working just on "physical" symptoms. All the time I was studying with her we were not working on parts but working to become more reactive altogether.[13]

In the 1930s and '40s in Germany there were intensely contrasting social and political trends; people were learning about the ideas of Freud, Marx, and, from Italy, Montessori, while at the same time Hitler was coming to power. Gindler was aware of all these things and demanded that her students be aware also. She stressed that the work they did in class should carry over into their daily lives, letting their awareness of their entire environment be sharpened.

Carola Speads, who studied and taught with Gindler, reports how Gindler's work developed beyond the perimeters of *Gymnastik* in a physical education context:

> What distinguished her teaching was her interest in the total effect of this work on the total person, not just the person's body. . . . What happened was not just correction, nor was it only education and improvement; basically a change of life-style occurred.[14]

Gindler, who was not Jewish, continued to teach during the Hitler regime, carefully avoiding any publicity, and did all that she could to assist people who were persecuted by him. She held special classes for Jewish students, teaching them how to deal with fear from a physical standpoint and how to maintain their strength in an extremely difficult time. She fed and housed Jewish students secretly in her basement, helping them find ways to regenerate new energy for survival instead of being psychically destroyed by their situation. Since her classes were open to the public, she had to maintain a neutral exterior, but her teaching reached those who needed it most. A student writes:

> Without compromising her students or herself, she also made extensive use of her classes for the purposes of resistance. It was known that new arrivals in the concentration camps were often ordered to stand erect whole nights through, and if they could not, were mistreated. In consequence, Elsa Gindler often did standing exercises with us. Without mentioning the purpose of such exercises, she helped us find out how we could stand longest and with the least strain.[15]

Gindler documented her work extensively. She had her students write reports of their experiments done outside of class. She also took photographs of students before and after working and wrote her own records as her work developed over 40 years. All this was destroyed when a bomb hit her studio just before the end of the war. She survived, but all of her records were gone, a tremendous blow to her.

Gindler continued teaching until 1960, and her work spread through Germany and into Switzerland, Sweden, France, Israel, and the United States during her lifetime. She trained a number of teachers, among them Sophie Ludwig, who now maintains Gindler's studio in Berlin, and Carola Speads, who now teaches throughout the United States and in Europe. Gindler may have been unknown to the lay person when she died in 1961, but professionals in the field knew of her work and of the wide-ranging effects it had in other fields such as teaching, music, psychoanalysis, and physical therapy.

Carola Speads

Speads studied with two other *Gymnastik* teachers before she met Gindler in the early 1920s. She writes, "As soon as I saw what she was doing I knew that this was exactly what I had always been striving for. From that time on I worked with no one else."[16]

Speads and Gindler worked closely together until Speads, who is Jewish, was forced to leave Germany in 1938. She and her husband immigrated to the United States in 1940, where she set up a studio in New York and called her work "Physical Re-education." She maintained contact with Gindler and went to Europe to work with her during several summers toward the end of Gindler's life. In an article written in 1977, Speads defines her work this way:

> Physical Re-education is the training of the conscious sensing of the body and its functioning. . . . The idea is to "let" the body and the parts of the body assume the positions which are natural to them, and let them function in their appropriate way. . . . The more the individual experiments and experiences and becomes aware of his body condition both at rest and in motion, the more he will become conscious of any changes, good or bad, and the more quickly he will allow or permit the body a chance to adjust to normal, if disturbed.
>
> Physical re-education is far more than a mere treatment of symptoms. Rather it is the discovery of how the body can be enticed to re-establish proper functioning . . . a technique for bringing about changes which affect the entire personality. Through its training in sensing, it helps re-establish normal functioning and gives the individual a way of meeting life less

helplessly. Life is more fun if you are not its victim but have the experience of mastery.[17]

Speads has written an excellent book, *Ways to Better Breathing*, which describes the attitude of experimenting, feeling kinesthetically what happens naturally in the body and allowing the breathing to go on without interference. We shouldn't look for one correct way to breathe, she says, but instead should make sure our breathing is adequate for what we are doing and that it is not restricted by mental or physical tensions. We can't change it by forcing a new pattern, but if we use "beneficial stimuli," as Speads calls it, in the form of simple breathing experiments, the breath becomes adequate on its own. The student might breathe through a straw, or sit in different positions to feel the breathing in the body, or do different types of gentle massage in order to encourage any interferences to dissolve. With Speads' book as a guide, one can try out the experiments and at the same time absorb the essential attitude of awareness work.

Charlotte Selver

Selver also trained with other *Gymnastik* teachers before meeting Gindler in the mid-1920s. She studied with Gindler until she left Germany and maintained contact with her until the end of Gindler's life. When Selver came to the United States in 1938, she gave the name "Sensory Awareness" to her work and gradually attracted the attention of several psychoanalysts and philosophers, such as Fritz Perls, Erich Fromm, and Alan Watts. The Zen community also responded to her nonverbal approach, with its emphasis on awareness rather than intellectual analysis.

In 1963, Selver began teaching at the newly founded Esalen Institute in California, and soon her work was widely known in all the interrelated health professions that focused on personal growth. In 1970, a foundation was set up to further Selver's work by publishing literature and publicizing classes and teachers of Sensory Awareness. Members of the foundation have made a great contribution to the documentation of awareness work through their ongoing research and publication of interviews, articles, and reports about the work that originated with Gindler. (See Bibliography.) Charles Brooks, Selver's husband and co-teacher, wrote *Sensory Awareness, The Rediscovery of Experiencing* in 1974. Selver now regularly holds workshops in California, New York, Maine, and Mexico.

Selver describes sensing or being awake as not only being fun, but

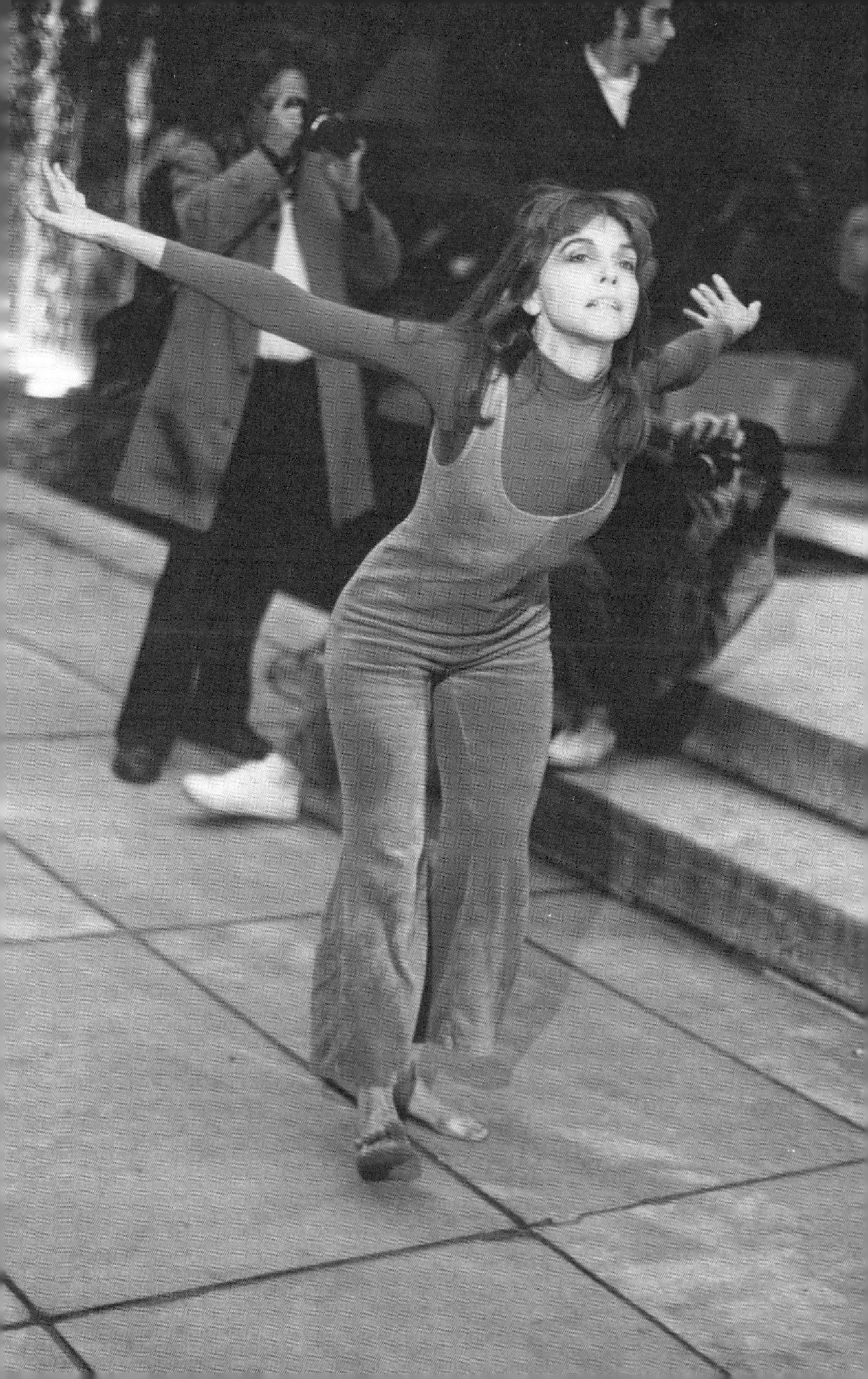

healthy. "Interest fires the tissue. Vitality, nerve activity, organic functioning, reactiveness are at their best, when we are really interested and in contact with what we are doing."[18] This kind of interest, or "direct perception," as she calls it, is contrasted with an intellectual or analytical way of approaching a task, the approach that unfortunately is stressed in both family and school learning. As Gindler also pointed out, the inward and outward senses can give us a wealth of learning experiences very directly, and by remaining available for these experiences we can make use of all our innate capacities. Our thinking minds can carry on without drowning our direct perception because they are two different functions, and we want to use them both. The essence of the Sensory Awareness work, says Brooks, "lies in distinguishing our actual experience from our thoughts and fantasies."[19]

Elaine Summers

Summers has made several important contributions to the developing field of awareness work, each of which will be discussed in some detail in later chapters. Being a dancer at heart, she values movement for its own sake and for its benefits to both physical and mental health. She states that Kinetic Awareness can be a beneficial basis for any dance technique, since it offers dancers the safety of truly understanding one's own individual instrument. She works with many dancers, as well as performers in other arts such as theater and music.

Summers has structured Kinetic Awareness into five phases (see page 30), allowing students to begin this potentially perplexing process of discovery at a manageable level. Her system of exercises using rubber balls (see page 41) as props and aids to increase awareness is a unique aspect of the work and one that has many advantages, as I will discuss later.

In addition, Summers always combines the subjective experiential process of sensing the body with an objective look at anatomy and physiology. Knowing the structure and function that we have, she says, can help us to use it fully and enjoy its intricacies. The goal of her work is to be able "to move every part of the body all the ways it can go, easily, any time you want, with as much or as little tension as you want, at any speed."

Elaine Summers performing "Energy Changes."

In 1968, as she saw her choreography incorporating more and more of the principles of Kinetic Awareness, Summers formed a dance company and began to train dancers over a three-year period. The company's first performance in New York in 1971 was the three-hour piece "Energy Changes," which uses the Kinetic Awareness principles and goals as choreographic structures. Summers also founded the Experimental Intermedia Foundation in 1968 to support and administer the work of several like-minded musicians, filmmakers, and choreographers. During this time Summers began to teach Kinetic Awareness to the general public, offering the first introductory course in 1968.

Since then the introductory course has been available twice each year, and Summers has taught many advanced classes, weekend intensives, and special workshops in New York and throughout the United States. Today, Elaine Summers continues her work, teaching privately on a limited basis. In recent years, she has also begun to train and certify a growing number of Kinetic Awareness teachers. While most certified teachers have remained in the New York area, Kinetic Awareness is beginning to spread across the nation. This year, under Summers' direction, the Kinetic Awareness Center has been established to promote both the teaching and wider practice of Kinetic Awareness. For more information on the center and on Kinetic Awareness teachers, see page 74.

Notes

1. Information about Elaine Summers and her development of Kinetic Awareness is taken from a series of interviews with Ms. Summers, beginning in 1981, as well as years of study with her as a student and teacher-in-training.

2. Janet Collins, Merce Cunningham, Jean Erdman, Martha Graham, Louis Horst, Daniel Nagrin, Don Redlich and Anthony Tudor.

3. Readers interested in a more detailed analysis of the work of Freud and Reich may wish to read *A General Selection from the Works of Sigmund Freud*, edited by John Rickman; *Selected Writings: An Introduction to Orgonomy*, by Wilhelm Reich; or *Bodymind*, by Ken Dychtwald.

4. Reich, *Selected Writings*, pages 109–10.

5. *Ibid.*, page 172.

6. *Ibid.*, page 144.

7. Brooks, *Sensory Awareness*, page 231.

8. Stebbins had studied with François Delsarte and Steele MacKaye, both of whom worked primarily in a theater context.

9. Gindler, "*Gymnastik* for Busy People," pages 36–37.

10. *Ibid.*, page 38.

11. *Ibid.*, page 40.

12. *Ibid.*

13. "Elsa Gindler Recalled by her Early Students," *Bulletin: Elsa Gindler 1885–1961,* vol. I, no. 10, page 29.

14. "Somatics Interview with Carola Speads," *Somatics*, vol. 3, no. 2 (Spring/Summer 1981), page 11.

15. Lily Pincus, "Lost, Won—My Way from Berlin to London," *Bulletin: Elsa Gindler 1885–1961,* vol. II, no. 10, page 33.

16. "Somatics Interview with Carola Speads," page 11.

17. "Physical Re-Education: What It Is and What It Is Not," *Somatics*, vol. 1, no. 2 (Spring 1977), pages 22–23.

18. Charlotte Selver, "Sensory Awareness and Total Functioning," *General Semantics Bulletin*, nos. 20 and 21, page 8.

19. Brooks, *Sensory Awareness*, page 201.

3

The Working Process

This chapter will introduce you to the scope of Kinetic Awareness work by taking you, as far as words can, into a teaching session. I have tried to provide a very close approximation of what you might expect and experience during your first lesson, as well as to review the basic working principles that form the core of the Kinetic Awareness process. Because it intimately involves the bodymind, however, Kinetic Awareness cannot be learned from a description, no matter how detailed. To make Kinetic Awareness your own, you must take the next step—study with a certified teacher. If you have already begun your study, I hope that this book will validate and clarify the journey that you have started and answer any questions that may come up during the working process. However, reading about the work cannot replace doing it.

The five phases of Kinetic Awareness

Once you begin study, your pace is entirely up to you. It is as individual as the bodywork itself. Summers has, however, divided Kinetic Awareness work into five general phases that will help clarify the progression that you can expect your study to take. Underlying these five phases is the real goal of Kinetic Awareness: the enjoyment and use of the bodymind's full capacity for awareness and movement. The five phases of Kinetic Awareness are:

1. The student learns to become aware of each part of the body, and to move each part by itself in all the directions it will go, as slowly as possible and with as little tension as possible.
2. The student can now articulate freely more than one part of the body at a time, slowly and without unnecessary tension. Students sense the constant activity of the body's all-over systems, such as the circulatory, respiratory, endocrine, and nervous systems, and how they interrelate. Slow movement using all the parts of the body simultaneously with minimum tension is practiced.

3. The student uses what was learned in phases 1 and 2 and now explores moving at different speeds, while still remaining aware and without unnecessary tension.

4. The student now learns to change tension levels at will through the entire scale from minimum to maximum tension, while maintaining the awareness and skills gained in phases 1, 2, and 3.

5. Movement through space and interactions with others are added. The student's concentration and awareness of movement articulation, tension levels, and speed are fully developed and can be maintained in performance, if desired.

As you might expect, most people work in the first two phases for several years. Many never go beyond that and still experience profound benefits. It is that part of the work that is the most different from most people's experience of their body. Even after all the phases have been experienced, the first-phase work is always valuable as therapy and injury protection. The beauty of this system of five phases is that at every level, the action to be done is simple and the goals specific, yet the effects are profound and complex.

Which step to take—private or group classes?

Although you can practice some aspects of Kinetic Awareness after only one or two sessions, the best way to begin to investigate its full range of possibilities for you is to take a series of classes. Your own understanding of the workings of your own bodymind will accumulate and the rewards will intensify over this initial period. The work can begin with private sessions or with a group in an introductory course that usually consists of a series of 10 to 15 classes.

Many students choose to take the introductory course and supplement it with a number of private sessions in order to work more thoroughly on their own individual body problems. I began work on my knee injury in private sessions, and when I saw the results, quickly went into group course work. Others take a series of private classes, continue work on their own, and then return for periodic sessions as needed. How you study, individually or in a group, is totally up to you, depending on your particular needs at any given time. As with so much of the Kinetic Awareness experience, there is no objective right way and no wrong way—there is the way that is right for you.

If you choose to work privately, the number of sessions each week and the program of study will be up to you and your teacher. One

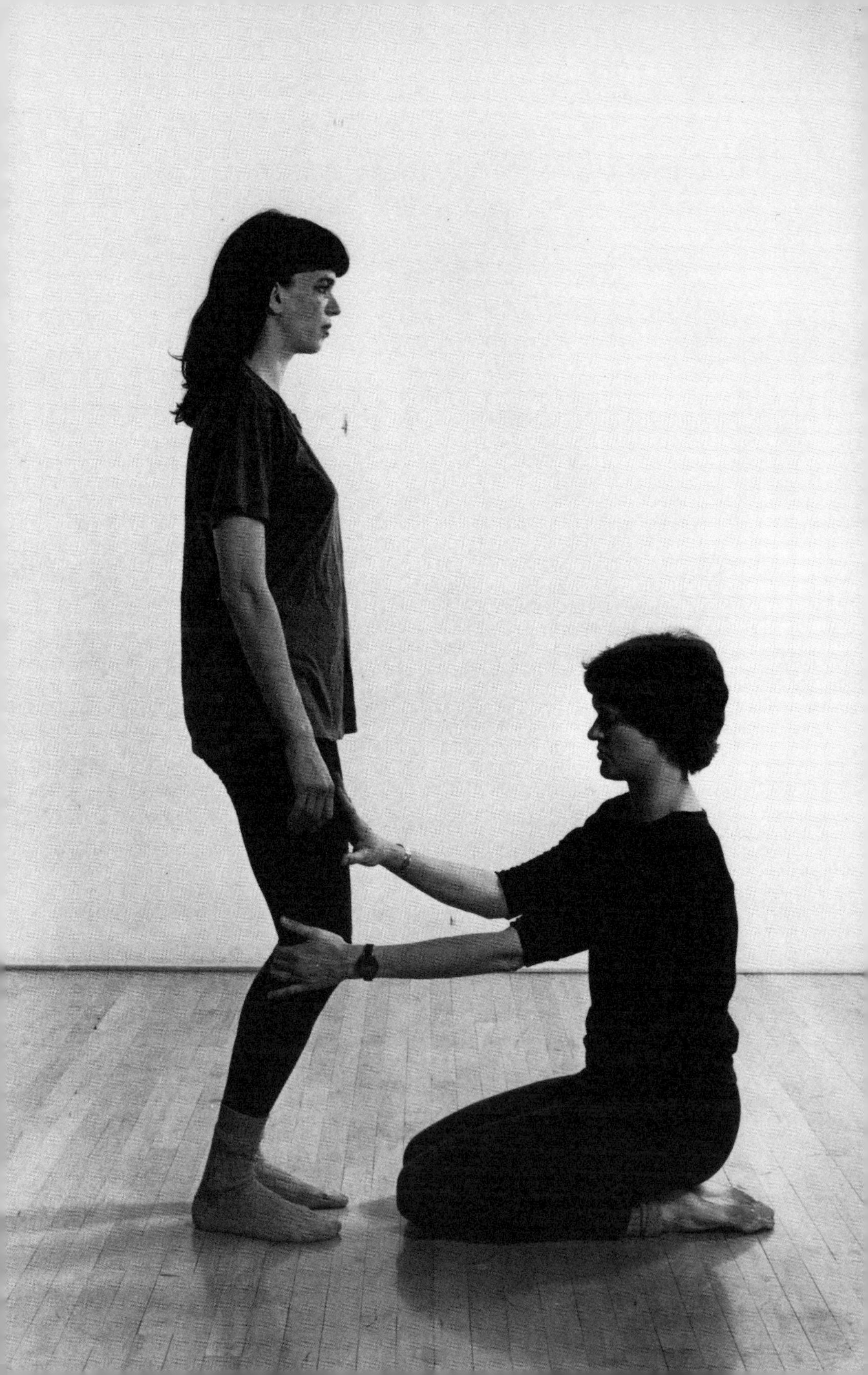

problem area can be the focus for several classes, using several different approaches to one body part, or the agenda can be varied in ways that are particularly appropriate to your needs. Some students prefer private sessions. There is more time for discussion between teacher and student, as well as more flexibility for the teacher to tailor what's being done based on the student's experience and reactions. Teacher and student also have more opportunity to form an in-depth view of how life experiences have influenced both physical and emotional health.

"In the beginning, when I was in a lot of pain, I wanted my teacher all to myself," Lily Besson, a writer, said recently. "When I grew more secure, when I was ready to explore other parts of my body besides my injured shoulder," she continued, "I looked forward to joining the group."

Many students look forward to group work from the beginning, however, and start with the introductory course. In each class, you are likely to find men and women of various ages and from various backgrounds who have come to Kinetic Awareness as a therapeutic treatment for particular injuries or chronic pain. Good news, as they say, travels fast, and beginning students often report hearing about Kinetic Awareness from a friend whose sciatica was relieved or whose headache disappeared after a few sessions.

Others come to understand and to explore their bodies. Many dancers and other performers use Kinetic Awareness to refine their expressive and technical skills and to protect themselves from injury, but it is open to lawyers, homemakers, nurses, teachers, physicians, accountants—anyone who is interested in learning about his or her body from an experiential point of view. Private sessions are often given as birthday or holiday gifts and lead to continued study.

Whatever the reason for beginning Kinetic Awareness study—and I sometimes think there are as many reasons as there are students—addiction to the work develops quickly. "If I can make one part of my body feel so much better by doing this," students say to themselves, as I said to myself over a decade ago, "why not work on each and every part—and feel great all over?"

The group, which is usually limited to no more than 15 students, comes together once each week to explore the part of the body that is the

In a private session the teacher and student work in detail on individual problem areas. (Caroline Simonds, left; Ellen Saltonstall, right.)

topic for that two-hour class. The sequence of topics may vary from one teacher to another and sometimes may depend on the characteristics and/or problems of the class members. My own standard sequence begins with the neck, because it is easier for new students to isolate, and continues in this order: shoulders, pelvis, lower back, chest, breathing, face, stomach, feet, knees, hips, and whole body.

A more detailed description of how a typical class might proceed will follow on page 45.

Working principles

Before you step into the studio, I would like to discuss, in some detail, eight basic principles that you can expect to encounter in Kinetic Awareness as you work with your teacher and on your own. They are awareness without judgment, learning to move slowly, using as little effort as possible, isolation, using tension as an ally, discovering the effects of breathing, using the rubber ball system, and the role of the teacher.

Awareness without judgment

Any Kinetic Awareness class, either group or private, begins with the very basic process of becoming more aware of the body, of beginning to listen to what the body has to say. This can be done in any position, but it is usually done lying on a thin mat on the floor so that students can close their eyes and concentrate easily.

For many people, it is a new endeavor just to observe how their body feels from the inside rather than how they think it should feel or used to feel—or even how it looks. The emphasis in Kinetic Awareness class is to have an awareness of the body right now, without the mind dominating, but feeling whatever is there to feel. Sensing the overall body position, the joints, bones, muscles, how they change during class—all these might be new observations of what we usually don't notice in our daily lives. We might notice that one part of the body feels stiff, another part feels comfortable, another part feels uncomfortable, and yet another part we can't feel at all.

It is important not to judge the feelings that come or to think that some are more important than others. Usually we are quick to comment, analyze, and judge the sensations of our body. Some of us have become used to noticing only unpleasant feelings as if when everything is fine, there is no need to pay attention to the body. Others suppress those bothersome feelings, the aches and pains, and notice only the pleasant ones. Both are worth noticing, because we can use that feedback to know how our body functions best. As we listen more to *all* the body's messages, we are fine-tuning that bodymind connection. We are allowing sensations to surface that may have been censored because of pain, our self-image, or our own fears of the body.

By being aware of the whole range of our sensations from the inside, we can choose how to use the body. When something feels good, we know that we are giving the body what it needs for good health. Or, as Tony put it, "Kinetic Awareness teaches you how to move, slows you down, and makes you see how everything is lined up. Where it all is, what it feels like."

Learning to move slowly

Any movements done in the first phase of the work are done as slowly as possible. Many beginning students are skeptical when I tell them that with practice, they'll be able to move so slowly that the movement will be invisible, and that the only evidence to the observer that they have moved will be the change in position after time has passed. Sections of Summers' dance "Energy Changes" are good examples of this extremely slow movement.

When we slow down, it is much easier to feel each part of the movement and notice all the accompanying sensations. Moving at an ordinary speed, such as we would when pulling on a shirt or lifting a dish, doesn't allow us to separate the many different sensations that accompany the action; it becomes a familiar blur with perhaps only the end result being clearly experienced. Very slow movements, however, can provide a universe of discovery. For example, before he knew about Kinetic Awareness, Tony often felt the need to slow down in whatever he was doing "to crystallize it," as he described it, "and see what it really breaks down to be."

Tom, who initially had difficulty with moving slowly, recalls that "it was the first time I'd ever thought about doing things in a small way or slow way. And the rightness of it struck me." He finds that the slowness helps him achieve a release of tension and gives him a new souce of energy. "It's as refreshing as a good long nap." Since Tom drives his cab eight to ten hours a day, five days a week, this is particularly important.

Moving very slowly allows us to see what happens in our body when we tell a specific body part to move. We see which parts move easily and which parts resist. We see how we prefer certain movements to others, and the slowness helps us to interrupt the automatic patterns and find a new way to move, one that perhaps extends our range.

Pauline Oliveros, a composer and musician, reports that "the slow movement was the thing that was most interesting for me, and liberating. The awareness through slow motion . . . the notion of the body moving itself; the involuntary mode, and how to get to that . . . so that what you're telling your body to do coincides with what's natural for the body to do."

Using as little effort as possible

In addition to moving slowly, we also try to move with the least possible muscle effort. How little or how much does it take to move a shoulder? Can we let go of unnecessary muscles that move only out of habit? Can we release the tension that we needed to move and really feel gravity's power as it pulls our shoulder back to the floor? You may feel the difference between moving by contracting and moving by stretching the muscles. You might also feel the difference between those times when movement is difficult and when it is easy, positions in which your body is working and those in which there is total rest. All of these discoveries will provide a closer connection between your analytic or intellectual mind and your bodymind.

Simple as they are, these slow movements may be frustrating to you, as they were to me when I began to study Kinetic Awareness. Many of us are accustomed to moving fast, or with all our efforts, or moving to create a certain visual effect (all of which are predominant demands in performance-art training). Internal focus may be a new experience, but it has its own rewards.

Carola Speads in her book, *Ways to Better Breathing*, describes the process of using minimum effort and its relationship to breathing, a topic I will take up later in this section. As she points out, its effects are often profound:

> Move extremely slowly and with the smallest effort possible. Feel yourself when moving. What, first of all, is the quality of your movement? What does it feel like? Moving so very slowly may make you notice that your movement began with an involuntary "startle" instead of slowly, as you had intended. You may become aware that it was jerky rather than steady, and that it was sometimes followed by collapse. Obviously these are features of a poor way of moving. Try to overcome these malfunctions; aim for slow, gentle, steady and flowing movements, executed with no more than appropriate effort. But even though your movements are not yet perfect, you will feel their stimulating effect on your breathing, as well as changes in

> your total body condition. You may yawn profusely, sigh with relief, draw fuller breaths, and feel your breathing spread vigorously through your trunk, particularly into the small of your back. At the same time you may feel the need to lengthen your trunk so that you can rest solidly on the floor.[1]

Isolation, or moving one part all the ways it can go

Another important aspect of Kinetic Awareness is isolated movement, that is, moving one part of the body by itself rather than pushing or pulling it with other parts. For instance, you can move your shoulders by moving your arms or your back, but you can also move them by very specific initiation of the muscles around the shoulder joints themselves.

Paul Schilder, in his book *The Image and Appearance of the Human Body*, writes:

> We do not know very much about our body unless we move it. Movement is a great uniting factor between the different parts of our body. By movement we come into a definite relationship to the outside and to objects, and only in contact with this outside world are we able to correlate the diverse impressions concerning our own body.[2]

By narrowing the field of attention, focusing on a specific joint or area of the body, you can sense more details about how you move and you can begin to recognize interrelationships. "When I began, I rarely moved my shoulders, especially my left shoulder, alone. My neck," Lily elaborates, "even my back wanted to get in on the act." Lily's injury exacerbated a habitual movement pattern established, at least in part, by her work at her word processor.

Just as Lily did, you will see which parts of your own body always want to join in on any given movement, and which parts prefer not to move much at all. As another student notes, even a small movement of only one part of the body can be a tremendous experience if that part has never moved before. Connected to this is learning to move each part of your body all the ways it will go. Summers maintains that if we actually were to do this on a regular basis, the muscles and joints would remain in a healthy, balanced, centered tone.

Each of us, however, has daily habits that favor certain movements, and our range of possibilities becomes reduced over time. Consciously exploring movement in all directions, not just the most familiar ones, becomes a process of discovery and a very therapeutic activity for the body as well. It wasn't until Lily began this phase of her work that her shoulder began to improve significantly.

Isolating a body part this way and moving it by itself is a skill that underlies a good, self-supporting *alignment*, that is, a balanced arrangement of each of the parts of the body in relation to the others. With sound alignment, you will have maximum strength and flexibility and be able to move easily, at will, with small adjustments exactly where and when they are needed to perform a particular gesture or task. This is the secret of good posture that allows safe, energy-efficient movement.

Using tension as an ally

The word "tension" is often associated with stress and has a negative connotation. But for Summers, tension is a wonderful part of the body's resources, to be used as needed. We need tension to move, but our muscles are able to work from 0 to 100 percent, and it is up to us to choose what amount of effort we want to use. When we use the appropriate amount of muscular effort for an action, we are working efficiently and will experience less fatigue. Using too much tension, however, will result not only in poor timing and coordination of movements, but also in residual tension that becomes "frozen" in the body if it is not consciously released. It is this "frozen tension" that Summers sees as a major cause of body problems and one that is thoroughly addressed in the practice of Kinetic Awareness. I will discuss it in more detail in Chapter 4.

The first and second stages of practice encourage us to explore the lower end of the tension scale in order to release frozen tension and to be able to make subtle adjustments rather than only large movements. You may find the slow, simple movements of the first-phase work agonizingly difficult, since muscles that are held in frozen tension are reluctant to move. Luckily, the work itself not only reveals the areas of tension but actually facilitates its release. This is one of the reasons that Kinetic Awareness work acts as a relaxation technique for many people. This relaxation is of a particular nature, however. As Genevieve Stabbins, whose work with the body was a forerunner of Gindler's, wrote over a hundred years ago:

> Relaxation is not to be confused with sluggishness, inactivity or indolence. Relaxation means being able consciously to be quiet within, and gain quiet, dynamic energies.[3]

This special quality of relaxation comes not from withdrawing energy, collapsing, or abdicating, but from a conscious attention to the amount of tension we want to use in the body. Gindler elaborated: ". . . relaxation is that condition in which we have the greatest capacity of reacting. It is a stillness within us, a readiness to respond appropriately to any stimulus."[4]

In class, you will begin by lying on the floor, in a centered, relaxed position. No muscle tension is called for in this position, but you may find, here or there, some involuntary holding. Often we resist gravity unconsciously even when we don't need to; we protect joints by holding them, even though it is movement that keeps normal joints healthy, not stillness. Now you may be asked to move some part of your body, your arm for example, away from the body's center. Since any movement we make is achieved by muscle activity, some tension will be required. You and your teacher will watch to see just how much. As you slowly return your arm to center, you actually practice releasing tension very specifically. This skill will serve you as well in day-to-day life.

By practicing this exercise of slowly putting tension into an area to move it, and slowly releasing, you attain the coordination to be able to choose how much tension you want and where you want to put it. Although it may seem paradoxical, the resulting relaxation is a very profound quietness that is also very alive and responsive.

You might want to try a simple experiment now, on your own. Do not change position from the one you've been reading in. Instead, close your eyes and ask yourself: Where do I feel tension in my body now? Where is it needed? What is it not? Where are my muscles contracted? For what purpose? Where are my muscles relaxed? If you're like many students, you may be amazed at what you discover.

Feeling your own personal tension pattern is the first step toward control of the whole range of tension available to you. Then, as you explore movement possibilities in specific areas, you have the chance to watch how much tension you really *need* to move, and if you are working slowly, you can gradually begin to release what you don't need. More effective than just lying still or sleeping, the slow movement serves to release tension because the mind is involved, watching and listening to sensations of the body and making choices about how you want to move. For many people, like Ray Harrell, a voice teacher, it's not the relaxation, but "the efficient use of energy and tension that's the goal" for both himself and his students.

Discovering the effects of breathing

There is an ancient Eastern belief that our lives are not measured in days, months, and years but rather by the number of breaths we take. Whether we share this belief or not, there can be no doubt that breathing is fundamental to life. It is for this reason that awareness of the breathing process is an integral part of all phases of Kinetic Awareness work. In the first phase, one or two classes will be specifically devoted to breathing work, and in each other area of concentration, attention will be called to the breath in order to understand what is happening in the bodymind.

Although our breathing is controlled automatically by the nervous system, it can be greatly affected and disturbed by physical and emotional stress. Most of us have felt out of breath after running, for instance, or constricted in the chest when we're scared or anxious. We may hold the breath while concentrating, or while doing a strenuous task. Our common interferences are usually forceful inhaling, such as gasping, or holding the breath during or before exhalation, as in grunting.

Sue, who is also a pianist, noticed how much her sense of musical rhythm was influenced by her breathing patterns; when she was anxious, or concentrating on difficult passages, her breathing would be unsteady and her rhythm askew.

It is natural for such changes in the breathing to happen. In some cases, changes in breathing can be beneficial—such as in childbirth or in running for a bus. But sometimes the disturbance, or change, in breathing remains after its initial cause has passed. These disturbances become poor breathing habits that we can unconsciously retain the same way we retain muscle armor or frozen tension. Breathing then becomes inadequate, stamina is reduced, we lose mental clarity, and the muscles don't receive as much oxygen from the circulatory system which carries it from the lungs.

Of course, everyone's needs are different and subjective; there is no one "right" way to breath. But we are most comfortable if our breathing is natural, easy, and steady, and if it can adjust to differing situations freely. This is definitely under our control, as Gindler described:

> In difficult situations—for example in marital quarrels or with the unexpected appearance of one's employer—we see that this gasping for breath and cramp in the diaphragm and stomach regions assumes frightening dimensions. Breathing stops, or a breath is hastily drawn, and the situation—which probably demands our greatest responsiveness—is hopelessly lost. We all know this condition well; embarrassment, anxiety, ill-humor, confusion in the mental and spiritual realms, trembling or an embarrassed fidgeting with arms and legs in the physical realm. If one is already conscious of how cramping—or constriction—can be eliminated by becoming aware of it, one is suddenly equal to the situation. The breath

> flows more freely, the mental confusion abates, one can make use of one's capacities.[5]

The first step in working on the breathing is just to observe the normal breath pattern to see if there are any interferences. Summers describes the process:

> Simply lie down and try to observe your breathing, which is very difficult. Try not to interfere with it. Try to notice yourself if you're interfering with it . . . how do you interfere with it? And what is the breathing like? Where does it come in? Where does it go out? What does it feel like? Where does it touch? Spend quite a long time just doing that, and then take your favorite deep breath. Why do you like it? What happens to your normal breathing after you've done it? Does it change it? Where do you feel it?

After watching the normal breath, students in a Kinetic Awareness class might do various breathing exercises or experiments. These are not prototypes of "good" breaths, but exaggerations of some part of the breath cycle as a means of letting the breath expand and improve on its own. Also, by doing something specific to the breathing process, students can feel the difference between the changed breath and the natural or usual breath. Tom is an asthma sufferer and has been for most of his life. During breathing work, he became aware of how much he held his breath when he was nervous. The greater ease in breathing that has resulted from his Kinetic Awareness work provided a dramatic relief.

The effects of working on the breathing can be specific or general, dramatic or subtle. The spine may lengthen, the shoulders and chest may relax, the voice may deepen, the mind may become clearer, the body may feel lighter or heavier. Whatever the response, easier breathing always brings easier movement and a greater feeling of well-being, since the breath is quite literally a foundation of being alive.

Using the rubber ball system

Kinetic Awareness is affectionately known to many as "the ball work," referring to the use of varying sizes of rubber balls to enhance awareness and release tension. While Gindler and others occasionally used balls and other props, Summers' approach is unique. She has developed a comprehensive rubber ball system—a system that I believe is a major contribution to the field of bodywork.

Although the balls are ordinary hollow or solid rubber toys that range from the size of a walnut to two feet in diameter, their importance to

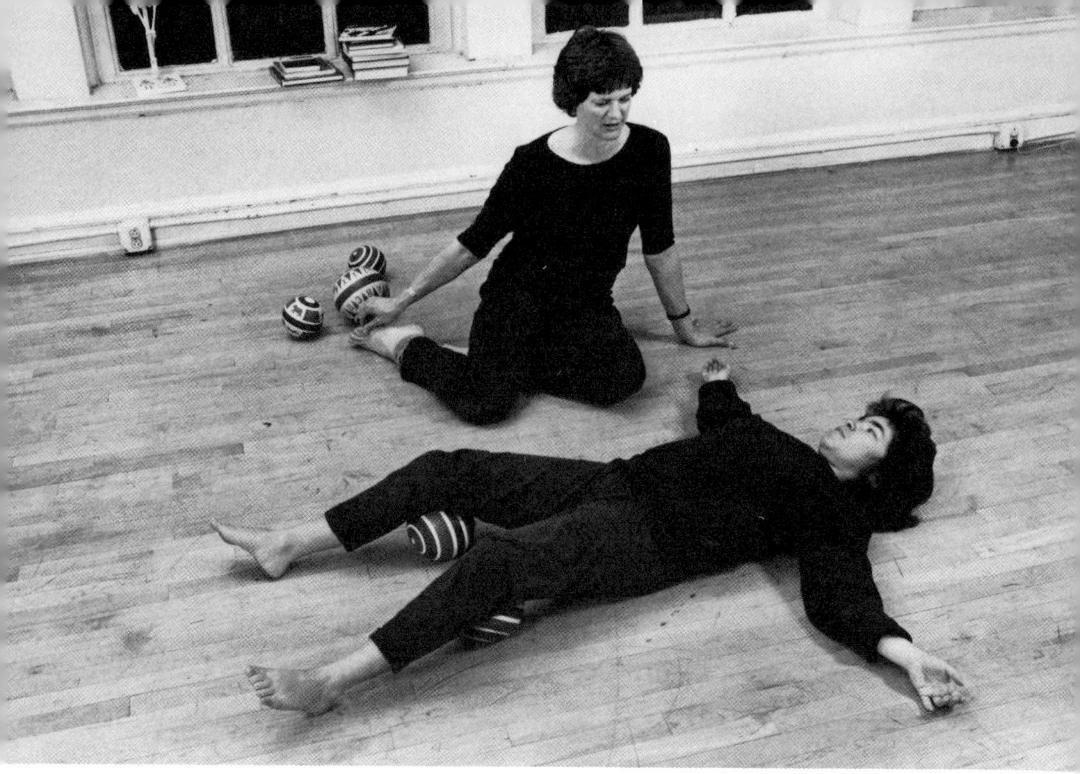

Hollow rubber balls of various sizes are used to focus sensation and movement on specific areas of the body. (Ellen Saltonstall, top; Arlene Greenberg, bottom.)

every phase of Kinetic Awareness work cannot be overestimated. They serve several key functions.

Beginning students use one ball at a time under one area of the body, then progress to using various combinations of up to five balls at once. The ball is placed under a specific area as a fulcrum for simple, slow movement. It provides a focal point, a clear reminder of where our attention should be, and it intensifies sensation in that particular area. Each small adjustment of the body on the floor can be felt vividly, with the balls as a magnifying glass for perceiving more details than one would in normal everyday motion.

Many students remark on this direct focusing quality of the ball work. Linda describes it as a "kind of depth probe," a nonthreatening way to locate trouble spots in her body.

By putting a ball under you while lying down and relaxing onto it, you are also getting a massage from its pressure. You can adjust the pressure according to your own needs and tolerance; a small or softer ball gives less pressure, a harder or larger ball gives more.

Rubber balls are used during almost every Kinetic Awareness class, especially during the first phase. Students may discover that as they move their bodies slowly and gently over the balls, they find themselves in new and unfamiliar positions. When this happens, students are often able to put their usual feelings and associations about their body on hold and thereby clear the slate for new learning to emerge. In general, they find themselves free to release habitual tension and to initiate movement with forgotten muscles, because suspension on the ball facilitates both. This can be particularly crucial following an injury. Lily explains, "by focusing on the ball just above my shoulder blade, I could 'forget' some of the pain in my arm and shoulder. Then it provided a sort of massaging encouragement that allowed me to let go of the tension that I had been carrying there."

Tom, who describes the ball as "a friendly tool," points out that most types of therapy can elicit anger against the therapist for trying to change deep-set habits, even when those changes are designed to help the patient. He appreciates the neutral and impersonal quality of the balls: "The balls are the closest thing to a gimmick, for a person who needs gimmicks, in a type of therapy that isn't going to permit a whole lot of gimmickry."

Learning to work with the balls with less tension translates easily into using less tension in other activities, as Tom, an avid horseback rider, saw right away. He found that he could drop his weight into the saddle better after learning to release his whole weight into gravity during class. As he learned not to press into the balls but to use them as a base for movement, his walk became lighter. He felt more limber in general.

Tom also points to another important aspect: balls are portable and easy to use, and most students find a myriad of uses for them outside class. "The balls are invaluable for things like traveling, just to prop my back up when I take a long airplane trip," he says. "It's like getting a massage from the inside. If I put balls under my thighs, or at my lower back, it's a much more comfortable trip. And it's much easier to drop off to sleep."

Summers has developed an enormous collection of ball-work exercises to treat virtually any body part or body problem. Each person will feel different sensations and notice different effects after using them. The balls help us to draw our attention inside, to listen to the body in a very intuitive way. Afterward, most people feel a pleasant quietness in both mind and body and a heightened sensitivity to movement and rest.

The role of the teacher

The Kinetic Awareness teacher fulfills a role different from the traditional one of instructor. People may come to a teacher wanting to be taught,

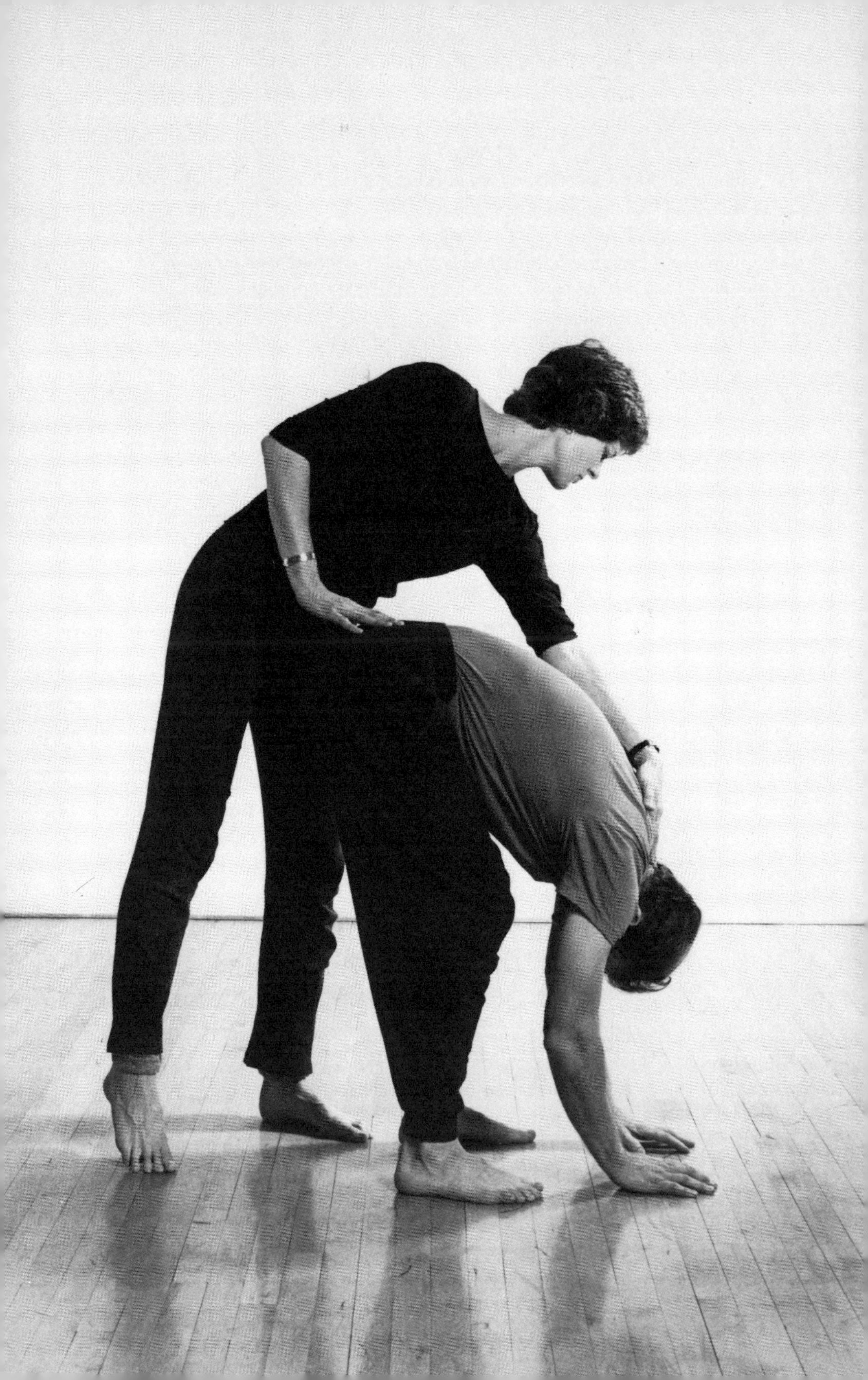

corrected, or exercised, but in Kinetic Awareness the teacher hands the responsibility for learning back to the student. He or she is more of a guide, helping the students to sense more of themselves by giving them simple situations in which to practice becoming more aware. There is much more listening and watching than teaching because the focus of the work is experiential and not intellectual. Your teacher will ask you questions, most often, "What to you feel?" He or she might also make observations relating to function or point out habits that often cause discomfort. Kinetic Awareness is an extremely practical approach. As Fenna describes it, "You look for the problem, its cause, and how to relieve it."

If a student is particularly reluctant to work on a certain area, the teacher won't force the issue or demand to know why the resistance is there. In other words, there is an acknowledgment that certain physical areas are highly charged emotionally, but there is no pressure to talk about private feelings; the teacher is not a therapist. The teacher's role is delicate but vital; he or she stands by, gives reassurance, and shows respect for each individual's way of using the body. The teacher doesn't manipulate or instruct a student to make certain discoveries, but sets the environment for a safe exploration. A natural and suitable pace is set by both teacher and student, respecting the wisdom of the body and not imposing specific standards or timetables. Kinetic Awareness "respects your own pace," is how Sue puts it, "and if you go by your own pace, you can't get hurt."

Some people experience profound changes in their bodies and emotions from the very beginning, while others feel the effects more gently. Neither experience is rewarded by the teacher, who is there just to support and facilitate each person's process of becoming more aware.

Description of first-phase work

Now that I've reviewed the basic principles of Kinetic Awareness work, I would like to "invite you into the studio" for a typical class.

In the introductory course, classes follow a simple format, varying slightly with each teacher and with the part of the body that is the topic of that particular session. Before the first class, or at the time of the first private lesson, I take a brief medical history—or, in the case of injury, a more extensive one—from each student.

The Kinetic Awareness teacher guides the student through simple movement sequences. (Ellen Saltonstall, left; John Milich, right.)

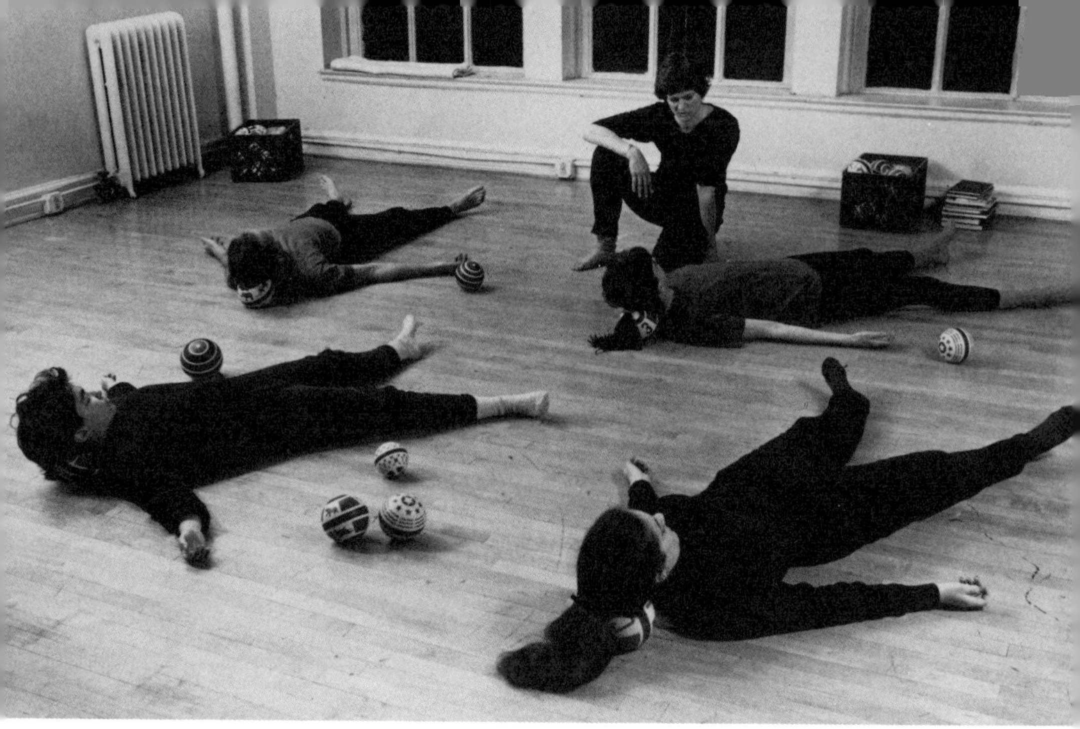

In this class focusing on the neck, each person works at his or her own pace, exploring movement over the ball with the neck and head. (From left to right: Arlene Greenberg, John Milich, Ellen Saltonstall, Caroline Simonds, and Marie Casey.)

The studio will probably look like a regular dance studio, with wooden floors and ample space for everyone to stretch out. Floor mats will often be used. The lights will be dimmed when class begins to diminish outward distractions and enhance concentration.

As noted earlier, the introductory course usually begins with a class devoted to the neck. You will start by lying on the floor on a mat, closing your eyes, and taking time to sense the entire body. As Summers points out, each day our bodies may feel quite different, and we don't know today's status quo until we take the time to let the body speak to us. You might feel quite peaceful, or agitated, or aware of discomfort in the back, or comfortable resting on the floor. The point is really just to notice how you feel.

After a few minutes, your teacher will call attention to the breath, and you will be asked to observe what it is like right now and how it feels. Then you might take a deep breath, sense that process, and see if it affects any of the other sensations already noticed. Each person in the class will be silently making entirely different observations, according to his or her own body.

Then you will begin to explore small, slow movements with the neck and head, moving in any direction that is possible but with minimum effort. It is important to initiate the movements from the neck itself instead of pushing or pulling with some nearby body part, such as the shoulder. Students sense the difference between active and passive movement; the neck is active but the shoulders, arms, or chest may feel slight passive movements. This is an exploratory time, with no particular goal other than to see what the neck can do, "as if you've never had a neck before," as Summers says. This movement exploration is done lying on the back and repeated while lying on each side and then the stomach, comprising about 20 minutes of the class.

Concentration on one part of the body moving slowly in this way is often difficult at first; we feel restless, frustated by reminders of sore and stiff muscles and joints. But at a certain point, the mind usually accepts the situation enough to enjoy, as Linda says, "doing something simple from the feeling state instead of mechanically." The inner workings of the body, the pitfalls as well as the pleasures, become a fascinating universe of discovery.

After this slow movement, you will be asked to rest quietly without doing anything to see if any sensations have changed simply by moving slowly and with concentrated attention. Usually, the neck will be more vividly felt. It may rest differently in relationship to the floor and the rest of the spine, and the breathing or some other body part may have re-adjusted, as Speads indicates.

Students then sit up to discuss their experiences. No one is required to talk, but many find it helpful to name physical sensations or emotional reactions that they experience while getting more in touch with their bodies. It is reassuring to hear other people describing similar feelings; sharing reduces the mystique of the body and our fear of what might be happening to us on the inside. We can see how universally similar bodies are, yet how unique each person is.

The next section of a neck class is spent working with one 5- or 6-inch rubber ball. At first you will place the ball at the very top of the neck, in the notch just below the skull. After spending some time getting used to the feeling of the ball being there and releasing the weight of the head into it, you'll begin to repeat the same slow movements. Now the concentration is on moving right from where the ball is, turning your head very slowly to the side or tilting it slightly to see what movement is possible and how it feels. After several minutes, working on this first spot, the ball is moved down an inch or so to a lower spot on the neck, and the same sequence of movement follows. This process continues for 20 to 40

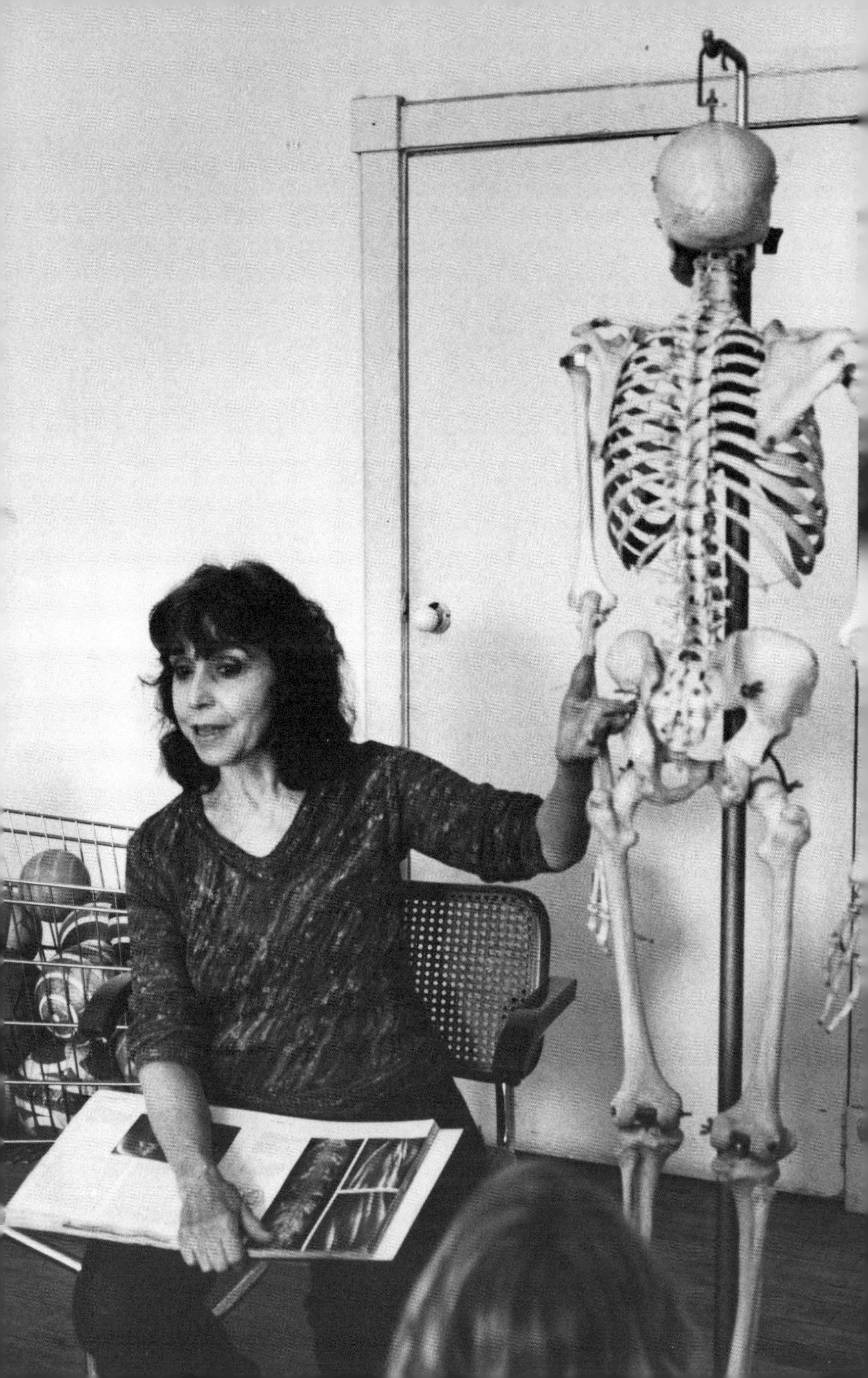

minutes. Then you will remove the ball from under your neck, lie flat on the floor, and see if you have any different sensations as a result of using the ball. Some will feel light, some heavy, some will feel much more relaxed, some will be more aware of tension areas because their total awareness is sharpened.

One again, students gather to share their findings. The teacher moves the class into a discussion of the anatomy of the neck: the bones, ligaments, muscles, and nerves that have been affected by that day's work. Pictures in anatomy books may be used for illustration, but the emphasis is always on making the connection between the factual structure and function as it appears in books and our actual experience as we sense our bodies.

Sue characterizes the subtle bodymind dialogue that takes place during this process. She reports getting "a much clearer idea of anatomy. . . . You can really feel how muscles change their shape, and you get to know yourself." This self-discovery, which takes courage, leads to an integrated mental and physical self-confidence, because, as Sue says, "by appreciating the complexity of things within you, you can really focus on what you have to teach yourself."

Summers feels strongly, and I agree, that this knowledge of anatomy is everyone's right—like having an owner's manual to the body. Many people have no access to this information in their previous education and have developed a fear of the body and dependence on doctors or others to help them interpret their physical sensations. Although experts are certainly helpful in many cases, we all have our innate "body wisdom" and can gain tremendous satisfaction from this experiential approach to anatomy.

If enough class time remains, students pair up to exchange brief massages on their necks. Massage can be an important part of the learning process, both mentally and physically. The person giving the massage can get a tactile understanding of the anatomical structures, feeling the bone and muscle connections, the various shapes and textures of the tissues. For the receiver, being touched can either mobilize insensitive areas or soothe areas that are tense, and it can give a shared feeling of support and reassurance. In fact, this support among students is felt all during the class, and changes happen more easily when students see and hear each other making new discoveries and shedding misconceptions about the body.

Elaine Summers discusses anatomy with students.

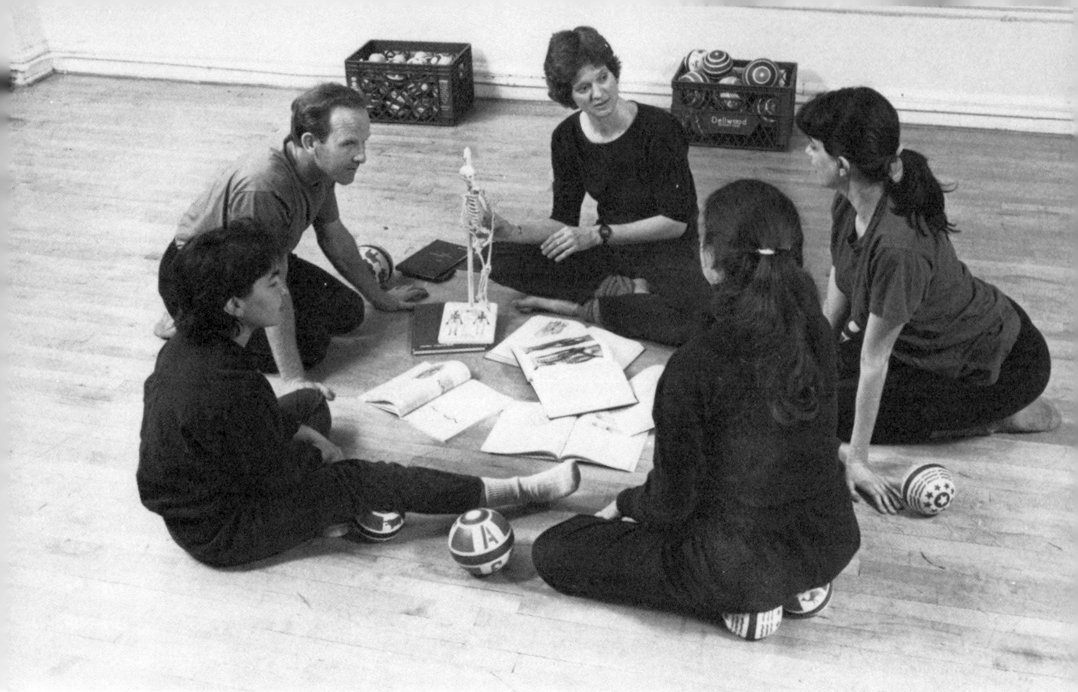

Discussion of anatomy with reference to illustrated textbooks and a skeleton helps to clarify the body's structure and function and relate it to the students' experience. (From left to right: Arlene Greenberg, John Milich, Ellen Saltonstall, Marie Casey, and Caroline Simonds.)

How the work is applied outside class

Summers stresses that maintaining awareness of our everyday movements has an essential and ongoing corrective effect. If we practice awareness only in class, we lose the opportunity to improve our body use in a meaningful way. The actions that we do every day are the ones that will provide the most appropriate "exercises" for improving ease and efficiency. Time spent with "on-the-spot" awareness amounts to much more than time spent in class. The principles and skills learned in class lend themselves to a continuous process of observation and application in daily life.

Students leave each class with both a slow therapeutic movement sequence to do for a specific body part and an "everyday action," or simple movement, that can be done anywhere and anytime to remind themselves to keep in tune with the body. For the neck, the everyday action might be to make slow, snake-like movements, easing up tension areas and very gently maintaining mobility. Through these everyday mini-awareness sessions, we begin to see the effects of our movement habits on our overall ability to move freely. Students describe the effects in various ways. Fenna reports that after working with Kinetic Awareness for a few months and getting relief from her discomfort, she began to

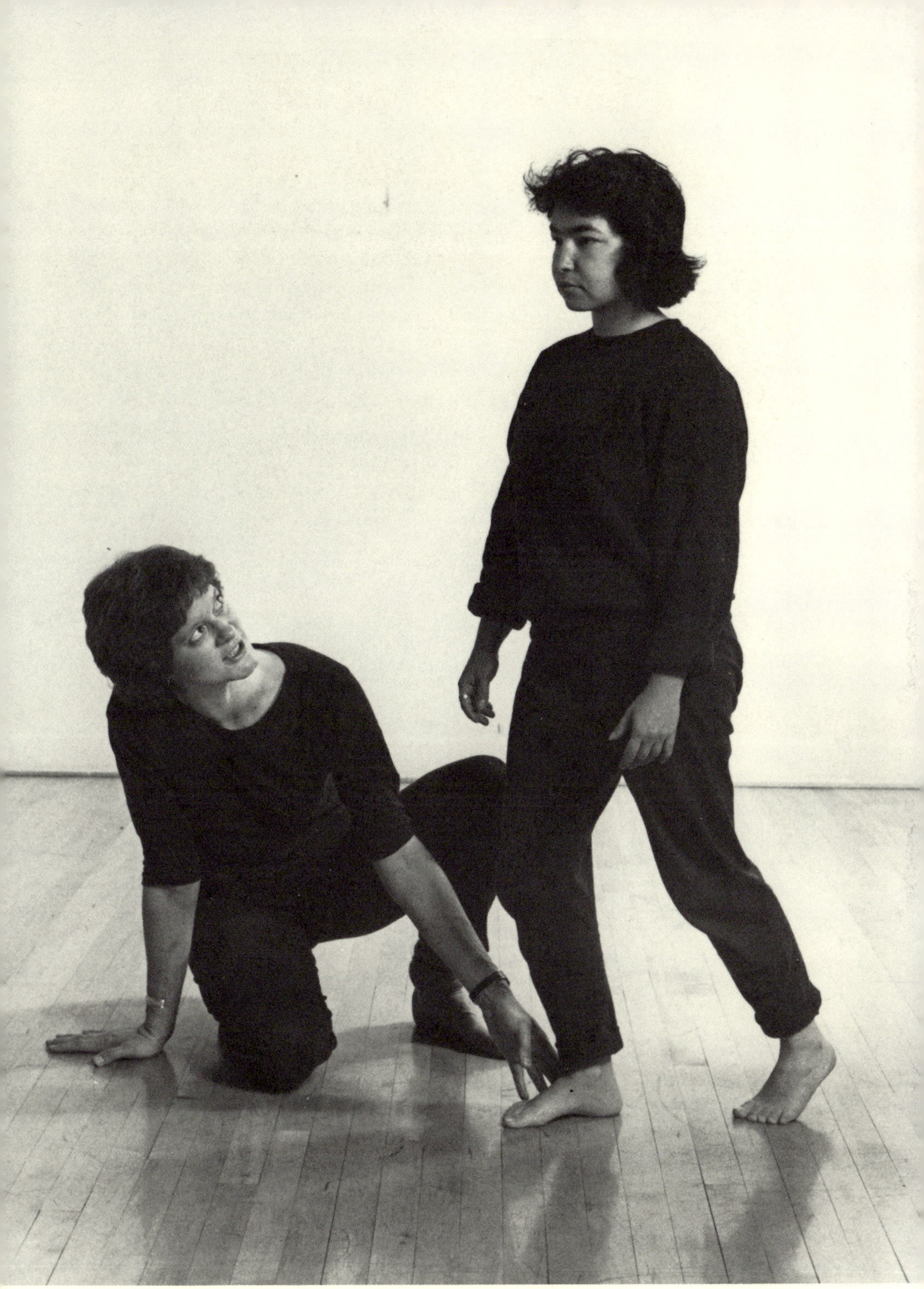

Everyday actions such as walking can be the focus of working toward a more finely tuned coordination of mind and body. (Ellen Saltonstall, left; Arlene Greenberg, right.)

notice ways in which specific tensions resulted from simple daily activities. She traced her hip tension to gripping in one leg as she pressed the brake peddle of her scooter; headaches seemed to be caused by straining to keep her eyeglasses from slipping off while doing housework.

Several people described how valuable it is for them to be able to do something at home on their own, to keep the work going between sessions. One dancer had had severe back problems that were not relieved by medical treatment. "It was clear to me," she said, "that when you do the work, it is a therapy that you can do yourself. . . . Once I was able to work with the balls, I had something I could do." She felt that in contrast to other techniques in which the patient or student is mostly passive, Kinetic Awareness gave her a sense of progress and independence, and it addressed her problem in a very active, personal way. Through intense work, her pain was relieved and she also gained a good understanding of what had caused the problem.

In a similar vein, Ray Harrell found that in his singing, Kinetic Awareness gave him a way of monitoring himself that other techniques, more reliant on the practitioner's touch, did not. While working on a piece of vocal music, he could put his head on a ball and play the recorded accompaniment, practicing this way until his body didn't react in counterproductive ways.

Anne-Reily Jones, a dancer and teacher, sees the work as a lifelong process, not just a classroom experience. She says, "The most important thing is really incorporating all those little things into what I do every day, whether it's watching how I stand to wash the dishes, or walking to school." Tony gained a kind of watchfulness for slight physical strains in daily activities so that he could take preventive measures before the strain became more serious by "just constantly changing to find a better way to do it." He found that actors often use excessive tension to get intensity into their delivery, and that this is really unnecessary. With Kinetic Awareness training, he says, "you need to use a whole lot less to get a whole lot more." Being skilled enough to change tension levels at will gives him "more color" in his performance. "Every single day of my life," he adds, "I'm reminded of this work, just by something simple like feeling my calf muscles stretch as I'm going down stairs. Kinetic Awareness is something that never goes away."

One dancer/choreographer I spoke with uses Kinetic Awareness as a training and preparation for her own particular style of dancing. Since her choreography is not based on a standardized technical vocabulary of movement, she and her dancers are quite reliant on what she calls a "very

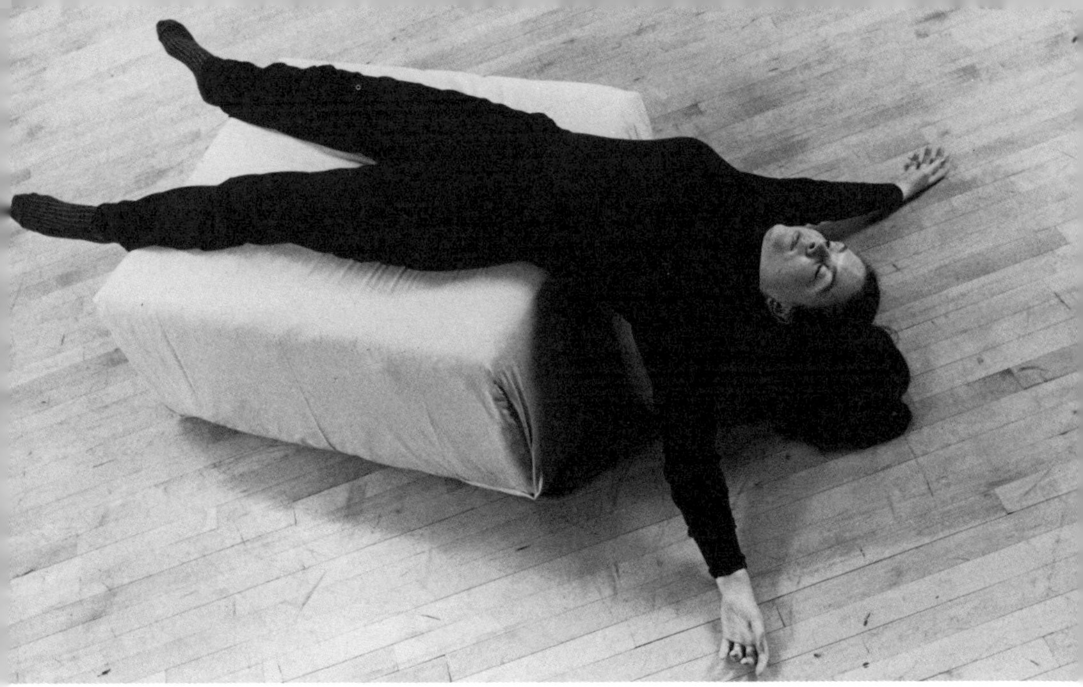

Marie Casey demonstrates how lying over a large foam cushion and a large ball gives an overall stretch of the spine and chest.

well-organized body," meaning a body whose movement is not restricted by habitual tension patterns but one that can make multidirectional shifts at a high speed. Using Kinetic Awareness, unwanted tension can be released and the body's all over alignment reasonably centered and ready for this type of movement. She predicts that as more dancers begin to see the body therapies as an integral part of their training and to see the work as preventative and educational in itself rather than just a therapeutic or "anti-technique," there will be a better breed of dancers and less of a dichotomy between technique and the body therapies.

Later phases of the work

Students always have the option of continuing the work in private sessions or combining private sessions with classwork. The later phases of the work build on the foundations formed by the slow, careful process described above. As more skills develop in areas of movement articulation, release of unnecessary tension, and breathing, students begin to also explore the conscious use of space, speed, tension levels, and interactions with others. After working on the floor with rubber balls, the focus turns to 1) simple movement sequences designed to increase awareness of the body's range and 2) opportunities to explore a complete range of movement through improvisation. Class format at this level can vary greatly depending on the interests of teacher and students, but the goal is to integrate the foundational skills into choreographed, improvised, and everyday movements. Often larger balls, two to three feet in diameter, and large foam cubes are used to assist the student in stretching along the whole spine.

One of the most frequent comments I hear in interviewing students is that Kinetic Awareness is a very "organic" method. A student soon reaches an acceptance and appreciation of his or her own body and mind and sets the pace and scope of the work, rather than following a prearranged format. Because of this, students become involved in doing the work for themselves, and it becomes part of their lives very naturally.

As Tony says, "To really personally put it into your body is something that takes a long time." The subtlety of the work, going back to a very basic inward understanding of bodily sensation and movement, is best understood in a gradual learning process over time, rather than one or two classes, he feels, because then it's a "constant exercise that goes on." When he did aerobic exercise he realized how much he relied on his Kinetic Awareness background to prevent himself from straining. He noted the danger of "anything that makes you move fast before you learn how to move slowly. . . . Kinetic Awareness teaches you how to move, slows you down, and makes you see how everything is lined up. Where it all is, what it feels like. And the second you start to feel bad, you have to be able to stop. Rub it, massage it, get off of it, take care of it, and then figure out: Why is this happening? They're not just fluke accidents, they build up for very specific reasons, and that's what it is, to try to learn that."

These comments lead to the frequently asked questions: Why and how do we injure ourselves? And why are our familiar body patterns so difficult to change? These questions and many others will be addressed in the following chapter.

Notes

1. Speads, *Ways to Better Breathing,* page 107.

2. Schilder, *The Image and Appearance of the Human Body,* page 112.

3. "The Development of the Concept of Relaxation in *Gymnastik,*" Ruth Norenberg, excerpted in Charlotte Selver Foundation *Bulletin,* vol. II, no. 10, page 21.

4. Gindler, "*Gymnastik* for Busy People," page 40.

5. *Ibid.,* page 38.

4

Physiological and Psychological Aspects of the Bodymind Connection

The very basis of Kinetic Awareness is to return to us our own natural bodymind connection. The method is very direct; by reawakening and sharpening our natural inner kinesthetic sense, we can use and enjoy the body for what it is.

However, during the process of working, many of our assumptions about our bodies and minds may be called into question. Many of us ignore certain parts of the body, for example, and close off sensations that might be clues to healthier movement. If the lower back or a hip or a shoulder is uncomfortable, we think we can pretend it doesn't hurt, and in time the pain may seem to disappear. We may not feel the pain, but perhaps this is because sensation in that area begins to dull. Movement becomes restricted, both because of the pain and because we choose not to use or even feel a troublesome joint. Perhaps we were taught as children not to pay attention to our bodies, not to give any importance to good or bad feelings, because our intellectual minds are more important. Detailed attention to the bodymind is often ridiculed as being narcissistic or hypochondriacal.

Unfortunately, when we don't listen to what our bodies can tell us, we gradually lose the skill; the messages soon seem faint or even disappear completely. Perhaps as adults we are scared, consciously or unconsciously, by the possible malfunction of the machine we call the body, the machine we may separate from our day-to-day awareness, the machine we may resent and sometimes wish we could replace. We are afraid we can't do anything about it, so we decide, again consciously or uconsciously, that it's better just to ignore the sensation.

In fact, our bodies are equipped with such sensitive self-supporting skills that a replacement could never be as subtle or as versatile. Our nervous system monitors every part of the body, registering many different types of sensations and providing every part of the body with potential for movement. All we have to do is to be attentive to the body and encourage our conscious minds to cooperate with the body's natural drive toward healthy functioning. Listen to the body's voice, in other words. Summers stresses that the body needs to move to be healthy, and this means not just some parts of the body, but *all* the parts. "The more you can get every part of yourself to sustain itself and move itself, the healthier you will be, and the less open to injury you will be," she says.

How do we learn to move parts that we have been ignoring or holding back from movement? By concentrating on our inner sensations in a particular part of the body, as in the Phase One work we discussed in the last chapter, we gradually can find out how that part can move and what feelings or messages it has for us. A little extra attention will probably tell us why that neck, lower back, or shoulder hurts. As we relearn the language of the body, we are getting back in touch with an innate skill that is always there for us. Restoring the bodymind's communication network takes time, quiet, and patience, but the rewards are great. Not only do tension and pain begin to dissolve, but we can move more efficiently. The feedback system between the brain and the muscles becomes clearer; our muscles learn to respond very specifically to our intentions. We gain alertness, coordination and ease in daily movements, and the pleasure of using the body with more clarity. Summers acknowledges that the work is a therapeutic process, but it can be much more:

> Everyone, for their life, needs to really explore their movement, what they can do. It's delicious and it's fun, and whether you're sick or healthy, it's an important thing to make a part of your life. We're beginning to realize that all of us have to move, and that it's something that happens all day long. So it's good to integrate it into your life, and enjoy this always available pleasure.

Causes of body problems

Students usually wonder how or why the body came to be the way it is—why they have the particular problems that they have. There are always reasons for the way we use our bodies—emotional, practical, and physiological reasons—and these aren't good or bad, they just are the composite result of who we are and what we've done. Problems such as chronic pain or loss of function can result from many causes: genetic factors, illness, cultural pressure such as conformity and competition, intense emotional experiences, or poor education, especially in dance and athletics. These problems remain because we ignore them or have no means to correct them. If medical help is sought, separate symptoms are treated more often than all-over causes.

Physiology

Starting at the very beginning of our lives, we are born with a specific genetic inheritance that includes basic structural body type, chemical balances within the body, metabolism, and nutritional needs. Some people have long legs and a short spine, some have a long spine and short legs, some have irregularities in their growth patterns, some have sensitivity to hot or cold temperatures or to certain foods. We are born with these characteristics and they influence the way our bodymind develops. For instance, I'm very sensitive to sugar and notice an unpleasant sense of both physical and mental fatigue after I eat it. Someone who is sensitive to cold might have a tendency to brace against cold temperatures with muscle tension. Those born with a bone or joint deformity, such as a club foot or abnormal spinal curves, will be affected in ways that will in time affect the way they carry their body weight and the way their muscular tension patterns develop.

Similarly, certain illnesses can cause a chain of aftereffects in the body that become compounded if they are ignored or not dealt with appropriately. Someone who has had polio, for instance, will be much weaker in the area of the body that was affected, leading to an imbalance in weight-bearing and movement patterns.

And as Summers also points out, "What you do every day in your life, your everyday movements, creates part of the geography of your body." Often, however, it is impossible to pinpoint exact causes and effects. Ken Dychtwald, in *Bodymind,* makes a similar observation:

> Walking, sleeping, bicycle riding, pounding nails, sitting, giving birth, and playing the piano are all activities that, regardless of their hereditary and psychoemotional components, serve to mold and shape our bodyminds. What we have done with ourselves, how we have done it, how frequently we have done it, and how it felt to be doing it are all reflected in the way we have developed our muscles, bones, and neuromuscular coordination.[1]

Frozen tension and body alignment

Far more common than genetics or disease as a cause of body problems is prolonged and excess muscle tension in our daily activities. When we are not aware of how to match our body's efforts to what we are doing, it is easy to build up inappropriate muscle tension, which can then cause secondary problems. It is in this area of therapy that Kinetic Awareness has the most to offer.

Muscles need to contract, to stretch, and to rest in order to maintain a healthy tone and to receive adequate nourishment from the circulatory system. If, however, a muscle is held in contraction it becomes "frozen," rigid, and immobile. Its blood supply is reduced, metabolic waste products such as lactic acid build up, and this brings more discomfort. Frozen tension can develop in any part of the body and remain there for long periods of time, causing a feeling of deadness, stiffness, or pain.

In addition to these localized symptoms, held muscle tension will also usually change the alignment of the body, or the way the parts of the body relate to each other and to gravity. When the body has good alignment, the bones support the body weight, the ligaments hold the bones in place, and the muscles are free for movement. However, if we always hold our head to the right, for instance, the muscles on the left side of the neck will try to compensate by becoming chronically tense. The effects of this, or any misalignment, can become quite complex as the other parts of the body compensate and movement patterns change because of restriction from the held tension. Not only is the resulting syndrome uncomfortable, but in order to hold the body upright, it robs the body of energy that could be used in movement. Most of the time, this is done unconsciously but quite skillfully. Usually, there will be a "scapegoat"; some part of the body will call out for help. We may think that this scapegoat is the only problem to work on, but usually there is a unique and complex tension pattern that determines our movement style. We soon see that we must be more observant of *how* we do ordinary things, rather than restricting *what* we do. The simplicity of the movement in the first phase of Kinetic Awareness shines a spotlight on the difficulties caused by our frozen tension; a movement we know to be theoretically easy can seem difficult or impossible if blocked by frozen tension. Together, the student and teacher of Kinetic Awareness start to look at all of the overlapping complexities happening in the body and to figure out what changes will make improvements.

Many of my students have come to Kinetic Awareness suffering from frozen tension. Lily came with a "frozen shoulder" that may have had its origin when she slipped and fell on the ice. Clara Jackson, a photographer, had a similar problem that may have been the result of carrying around heavy camera equipment without regard for her body's alignment and natural balance. Both women found relief through Kinetic Awareness work. Added body awareness led Clara to balance her equipment more carefully when she carried it.

Tom found that using Kinetic Awareness skills, he could monitor the amount of tension he needed in different situations and stop himself from habitually using more energy than he needed. By choosing how much was needed for a particular situation, he was able to improve his horseback riding technique, relax more while driving his cab, and reduce the frequency and intensity of migraine and asthma incidents. The key was to be able to observe and recognize his daily stresses and, through Kinetic Awareness, to counteract the tendency toward muscle tension.

A common way in which muscle tension can build up inappropriately is by a lack of proper warm-up. We need to prepare our muscles and joints adequately for any strenuous activity that we do, be it lifting, aerobics, dancing, sports, or mountain climbing. There are many ways to warm up, but the basic principle from Kinetic Awareness is to start with the muscles as relaxed as they can be and then move them carefully through their range of motion, increasing the force applied and the speed very gradually. This simple guideline has far-reaching application in training for dance or any other physical discipline. Warmed muscles can work efficiently; without warm-up, the body desperately tries to meet the demand and excessive uneven tension results.

Another important aspect of warming up the body for any activity, and one which is inherent in the first phase of Kinetic Awareness, is the idea of doing only what you are intending to do, and not something else as well. When we consciously move specific parts of the body by themselves, we avoid the situation of pitting some muscles against others. Many standard stretching exercises are done by using forced leverage from opposing muscle groups, but if we extend and stretch the muscles on their own, we can move with more finely tuned coordination that is quite delightful. Summers teaches that we can move most efficiently by using muscles "that will stretch you there." After practicing this with simple movements in class, students are often surprised by how good it feels to move this way.

How the mind shapes the body

Subtler aspects of the bodymind are those in which the mind shapes the body to fulfill its needs. At the psychological level, we are constantly translating between the body and the mind, sometimes consciously, sometimes unconsciously.

From birth onward we learn about ourselves in relation to the world by watching those around us. We learn to talk by imitaton, we learn skilled movements by imitation. Thus parents usually pass on their particular "body" style to their children, for better or worse. As children we value what we learn from those who are dear to us, so the patterns become deeply embossed. Family photographs are a gold mine for studying how physical makeup, traits, and habits are passed from generation to generation. We might see our daughter's stance reflecting our grandfather's. We might also discover photographs of little girls imitating the fashion model's slouch or little boys assuming the stance of John Wayne, for as we grow up, we also adopt the manners of our role models. Some stay with us for many years to come.

Laid onto this groundwork of bodymind development are other ways in which the mind can actually shape the body. As Wilhelm Reich pointed out, any physical action that is endowed with strong emotional import can be frozen into the body in the form of chronic muscle spasm, or muscular armor. Armor forms as a protection against some kind of unsatisfied urge for expression or as a defense against real or imagined danger, and once it is formed, it becomes invisible emotionally. But as we begin to unravel the clues in the body, these areas of armor will begin to release their emotional contents, which can be strong and unexpected. For example, Sue found the work to be quite an emotional experience, with a variety of feelings that range from sadness, fear, and anger to a playfulness and joy from working closely with the body. She also has found that bodywork is useful in unlocking repressed memories.

Whatever is released will be unique to the individual, and the role of the Kinetic Awareness teacher is to be a supportive listener. The tension pattern and its emotional counterpart may be released very quickly once it has surfaced, or it may not; the important step is for us to become aware of these bodymind connections and more accepting of our own special makeup. Charlotte Selver describes how she learned to understand her body's language:

> At times my holding back . . . was like a reflex. I said "No," as I had said it as a child, when I was forced into things I did not feel like, when I was pushed around, when I was interrupted and called away from what interested me most at the moment. Then I was only conscious that I said it; now I felt, my whole self said it, my "body" spoke. I suddenly realized that this tension was not "wrong," as I had always thought, but was the most honest expression of my real self.[2]

The understanding about what the body is doing, and why, must come from the student in an experiential way, not from the teacher. As Elsa Gindler wrote:

> The most essential things we have to keep in mind are: that any correction made from without is of little value, and that each of us must try to gain understanding for the special nature of our own constitution in order to learn how to take care of ourselves.[3]

Our body image

Besides our actual physical activities and their emotional legacies, the other main contributor to our body geography is our own personal body image. We may have an idea about how our posture should look, how our walk should look, or how our head and arms should move. For instance, we may prefer to think of ourselves as very strong by maintaining a straight, tight back, or as very humble by folding in the upper torso, thus expressing a valued personality trait through the body. We may think of ourselves as being too fat or too thin, and this will affect how we move. There are also cultural stereotypes that tend to group some types of posture and movement style as masculine, others as feminine. All of this, plus the influence of family and friends, mixes together and we create a composite body image of the way we think we are or wish to be. If our body image allows for the types of movements we ask our body to do, then all will be well. But usually there are some battles going on: the straight, stiff back is fine for standing tall, but it may balk at carrying heavy loads, or even bending to get into the car. Thus a student of Kinetic Awareness will notice right away, and throughout the working process, that the thinking mind can easily restrict movement possibilities just by creating a complex body image.

One of the first things to learn is that we *can* distinguish between real physical sensations and those dictated by thought or images. Selver's "direct perception," described by Brooks in *Sensory Awareness,* refers to the same process, which is to learn to use the kinesthetic senses for immediate physical feedback from the body. Anne-Reily relates a discovery about her body image. "One of the things I found through the Kinetic Awareness . . . when I was working on the balls, is that contrary to a former conception of myself, I am incredibly mobile." Lily found that although she had always believed that she had good posture, she discovered that she had a tendency to hunch her shoulders. Clara discovered to her amazement that she favors her right side over her left; this was not the body image that she had of herself when she first began to do Kinetic Awareness.

Sometimes these discoveries come easily, sometimes not so easily. If the emotional associations we have with certain body characteristics are strong and dear to us, they will be held more firmly by our bodymind than those we picked up casually on our way. The nonstructured exploratory approach of Kinetic Awareness provides a safe environment to allow changes to happen as we are ready for them rather than according to a sequence set by the technique or the instructor.

Effects of previous training

Another way in which the mind forms the body is by setting standards of right or wrong. Ideally, as children we explore freely, using our bodies without censorship, because the urge to explore permits movements of all kinds. Then we begin to be told that there is a right way to do things, and our attention becomes, as Brooks describes it, "divided between what we are doing and whether we are doing it right. . . . We are not able to give our attention fully; there are too many whispers of conscience distracting us."[4] Dancers and athletes are particularly prone to this attitude, since their training is full of do's and don't's. Certain sensations and certain movements become preferable to others; it may feel "wrong" to stand on the outside of the foot, or to relax the stomach muscles when they're not needed. Dancers and athletes make enormous investments of time and money in their training, and the effect of that training on the mental filtering of physical sensation should not be underestimated. The challenge, then, is to find the distinction between movement habits that have developed, our actual sensations, and our intention, or what we really want the body to be able to do. As Summers says:

> Everybody's body is their instrument, not just dancers. You've had this body all these years, and no one ever said to you: Why don't you go in a room and find out what it'll do? Why believe everything everyone tells you? Find out what's comfortable, what you like to do.

The same exploratory attitude applies to Summers' theory of how to deal with injuries.

Injury rehabilitation

Many people come to Kinetic Awareness for help in recovering from injuries of all types: falls, accidents, and especially the "wear-and-tear" type (sprains and strains) that often allow some functioning, but with pain. Summers has developed a rehabilitation program that has proved extremely helpful both in facilitating physical healing and in removing the sense of panic and helplessness that most people feel when injured.

Her first rule is to give attention to the injury as soon as possible after it is noticed. Consult the appropriate physician to determine what is injured. A qualified teacher can help you to sense in which ways the injury affects your bones, joints, ligaments, muscles, tendons, and nerves. This data collection is an important step toward consciously aiding the healing process, because when we know all the effects of the injury, we can adjust how we use the body in order to facilitate healing.

It is also important to keep the body weight off the injured part. Massage is often helpful, varying from a light massage to stimulate circulation and prevent excess swelling to a deeper one to prevent muscle spasm and stiffness. Summers recommends elevating the injured part whenever possible, and resting until the pain has subsided enough to use the part gently. However, healthy parts of the body should be kept moving as much as possible, so that unnecessary stiffness and atrophy don't compound the problem.

When movement of the injured area is possible without pain, moving it is the most therapeutic thing to do—as it is for noninjured bodies as well. Movement can be done passively, as when someone else gently moves an injured ankle or shoulder, or actively, but still without any weight on the injured part. Not only does movement increase circulation and sensation in the area, but it helps the muscles stay relaxed and responsive. Gradually the movement range and intensity can be increased, building strength until normal functioning is restored.

In some cases, ball-work exercises are used to rehabilitate after an injury, but in other cases the balls are not helpful. It is important, Summers believes, to see each injury as an individual set of circumstances and to devise ways of working that feel good. This way we can have the satisfaction of doing something for ourselves, of seeing progress day by day, and of helping the body's innate healing powers to do their job.

Acknowledging the bodymind

"The more I do the work, the more I am constantly amazed that the mind and the body are the same," Anne-Reily says as she begins her summary of what she's learned from Kinetic Awareness work. "You can separate them," she continues, "but if you do, it's self-destructive. It's all part of a total process. One time, the mind discovers something, the next time the body . . . it just unfolds." After suffering chronic depression for many years, Anne-Reily decided to try approaching it from the bodymind rather than through psychiatry. Awareness without judgment and a fresh look at her body image lead Anne-Reily to a new acceptance of herself. "Instead of trying to monitor and control who I am and what I want to be, I have become more accepting of just who I am. . . . I'm very aware of being much happier, and much more out in the world, and I know a lot of it is because my body is not so locked."

Several students have remarked to me how they are more in touch with their intuition through doing Kinetic Awareness. The body's wisdom speaks not only to the issues of the physical world, but to other aspects of their lives as well—their work, their relationships. As skills are learned that give the body more flexibility and articulation, the mind learns from that experience and becomes more flexible and articulate also. The body is the most direct place to start, because we have total access to all its capacities. We can learn to trust the body's feedback, which gives us a foundation of independence that is one of the hallmarks of Kinetic Awareness as a bodywork technique. As we are working, we are concentrating in a way that is open to both sensory and motor feedback and that presupposes that choices and changes can be made voluntarily and directly. Body and mind have equal say in the discussion. We can still go to others for help, but tapping our own vast potential becomes an adventure in itself.

When Ray Harrell directs opera, he notices that most young singers are used to being told what to do instead of being required by their teacher to explore for themselves the whole range of vocal and musical character elements. He sees Kinetic Awareness as an effective way to sensitively reduce the rigidity that comes from less-than-holistic vocal training. Using Kinetic Awareness as a techinque with his students "to remove conditioning in relation to voice," he says, "my emphasis is on developing the voice and acting technique. The awareness work is a means to that end. My reason is not therapy in any sense. My reason is technique. . . . I work to develop their technique through consciousness. . . . Technique, for me, means the ability to manifest whatever you need, to express the energy that's coming through you at the time. I see Kinetic Awareness as a tool toward the development of the individual and the consciousness of the body as an instrument."

Because a singer's repertory comes from many different historical periods, the styles of singing that are called for can vary tremendously, and singers need to be extremely versatile. To help his students in that direction, Mr. Harrell takes an interesting approach. "I have to work out a way in which they can find their way into all those places. . . . Which means that they have to be able to go back in history to the kinds of psycho-physical feelings of the people of that time, in that sound-scape, in that relationship to gravity, movement, trains, cars, cement. . . . That was a whole different time, so I have to help them find that time in their bodies, in order to be expressive of the music of that time. That's what I use the awareness work for." In the attempt to find a truthful emotional expression through the music, he has his students find the emotion inside themselves, through the body.

He goes on to say, "I have great respect for the depth of Kinetic Awareness, the depth of each individual, actually. Because that to me is what the work is about. It's about your own internal systems, how to balance them and to get what you want, and to be responsible and make choices."

The process of discovery that takes place during Kinetic Awareness is so fascinating that students often feel dramatically different after the first session, both physically and in their attitude toward the body. The finely tuned coordination and awareness that develop from the work bring a feeling of self-sufficiency, both mentally and physically. As changes begin to happen in the body we see that we don't need to be locked into poor posture or strained movement patterns; if the mind is willing, the body can change. Or, to be more specific, if the body's need to change is heard by the bodymind, then change will be possible.

A pleasurable ease comes from knowing that we can relieve aches and pains, learn about how the body works, and find our own healthy movement patterns, instead of having to depend on someone else's expertise for these things. As we become more familiar with each part of the body, its sensations and its movement possibilities, we see that we can adjust the carriage of the body weight to promote the greatest ease in the muscles and joints. Each part can move itself and protect itself from strain because of the feedback between mind and body. The uncovering of this innate bodymind collaboration is just as gratifying today as it was earlier in the century when Elsa Gindler wrote:

> The student begins to feel that he is in charge of himself. He suddenly feels that if he wishes he can work on his whole body in the same manner he worked on his shoulder girdle. His consciousness of self is heightened, he is no longer confused by the range of subject matter, he is encouraged. This is a state which cannot be attained by exercise alone, regardless of how thought-out it may be.[5]

Notes

1. Dychtwald, *Bodymind,* page 20.
2. "Beginning of Beginning," Charlotte Selver Foundation *Bulletin,* no. 2, (Spring 1971), page 6.
3. Gindler, "*Gymnastik* for Busy People," page 40.
4. Brooks, *Sensory Awareness,* page 232.
5. Brooks, *Sensory Awareness,* page 72.
6. Gindler, "*Gymnastik* for Busy People," page 37.

5

Kinetic Awareness as Education and as Therapy

Holistic systems for bodymind reeducation and personal growth clearly have a place in the frameworks of both education and health care; in fact, they bridge the gap between other systems such as traditional medicine, psychotherapy, and fitness programs. By participating in any of the systems, but particularly in Kinetic Awareness, one can gain new information and understanding about his or her bodymind, relieve pain, improve body use, increase mental and emotional clarity, and have a good time of it, too. I hope I have suggested in the preceding pages the full range of benefits that are readily available and directly applicable to anyone who comes to bodywork. In this chapter I will review and summarize these benefits.

It would be nice to be able to prove scientifically that bodywork really achieves its goals, but the success rate of this type of education or therapy is nearly impossible to quantify. This is because the effects are so broad-ranging. In addition, the participants come to the work from such varied backgrounds. Although groupings could be made according to types of pain or complaints, this would belie the fact that emotional history and outlook, as well as attitude toward the work, play a huge role in determining how the process will unfold. Causes cannot be pinpointed in many cases, and the variables are too numerous. The work must be validated by the experience of its participants and by the growth of its popularity.

The special qualities of the holistic approach

Because our culture as yet does not support an ongoing study of bodymind functioning, most of us find ourselves overwhelmed by our own confusing array of tensions, attitudes, and behaviors. We often don't know which aspects of ourselves most need to improve in order for our lives to improve. Elsa Gindler, and those who followed her, saw that this quandary could be solved only by a holistic approach that acknowledged that emotional, intellectual, sensory, and movement aspects of our being are all inextricably interwoven. I think that an analogy quoted by Edward Maisel in the introduction to his collection of F. M. Alexander's writings is particularly apt: working with the whole bodymind is like cleaning up a messy room in order to find a lost object rather than simply looking for the object amid the mess.[1]

The holistic approach may seem indirect, but it offers many advantages. Maisel's unidentified source continues:

> "The indirect way . . . may take a little longer, but it is more certain, will render further losses less likely, and will have accomplished something useful even if the missing object remains unfound. Also it may happen that something lost long since and which has been forgotten may turn up. It has, too, the further important advantage that one will at last become fully aware of the contents of the room in a way that one had not been before."

As therapy, the holistic approach of Kinetic Awareness is sure to give a student relief of symptoms and less likelihood of recurrence. Problems that have been ignored, such as poor sleep or digestion, are often affected. As education, Kinetic Awareness definitely increases self-understanding and unfolds potential; the "contents of the room" become clear and available. We learn the extent of our full range of physical motion and the many connections between our mental and physical selves. The work provides a context for in-depth discoveries that can relate to all aspects of our lives.

Aileen Crow is a therapist and a teacher of Alexander technique, another well-known bodywork system. She consulted Summers because of a persistent problem with her feet, felt immediate results from the work, and has integrated both specific and general ideas from it into her teaching. "This is a process of observing yourself in a lot of situations and finding out what it is that you do," she says, "and then knowing that you have choices about what you do. I feel that everybody can learn to work for themselves, and that's a real adventure."

Making connections and sharpening our kinesthetic sense

How does the bodymind integration occur in Kinetic Awareness? In contrast to other methods that call for specific mental processes in relation to the body or that are more goal-oriented, Kinetic Awareness allows for "mind" work on several different levels. We can choose to physically "feel" the anatomy, or we can physically "feel" our emotional selves in the body. We can approach it as a technique to be mastered, as a playful journey, or as a sensuous indulgence to be enjoyed. We can become absorbed in sensation and exploration, or we can quietly attend to the simple movement tasks and watch the results.

Some bodymind techniques require that the students discontinue their poor movement patterns or habits before more appropriate possibilities are attempted. Kinetic Awareness work lets the good and bad habits pass each other on the road, acknowledging once again the value of making conscious choices while working. Changing one's mechanical functioning, and concurrently one's mind state and body image, becomes a flux more than a prescribed sequence. Instead of having to inhibit old patterns by will, the Kinetic Awareness student has the help of the balls, which can alter familiar sensations enough to circumvent habitual movement. Reliance is less on the teacher's analysis and more on listening to what the balls and the body have to say. Because Kinetic Awareness can be both analytical and sensual, both affirming and corrective, it offers a richness and adaptability to many types of people.

Another advantage of Kinetic Awareness is how it focuses us in the present time. When preoccupied with outward responsibilities, many of us don't give ourselves the chance to "update" our awareness of our bodies. We remember how we felt last week after playing tennis, or how we felt yesterday after dance class, but we don't take time to be aware in an ongoing way. By constantly asking, "What do you feel now?", the Kinetic Awareness teacher reminds us to sharpen our kinesthetic sense and helps us to go beyond the limitations of our body image or our fears of pain by just observing what is there now. We learn to connect the anatomical information that our intellectual minds receive and process with the sensations that our bodies perceive and process. Information is gathered from many sources (sensations, observations from the teacher, touch, and movement), all of which removes the usual mystery surrounding how the body works. Being connected in this way, without a sense of right or wrong but with "unprejudiced conscious attention,"[2] we can remain in touch with our constantly changing physical and mental states.

As our kinesthetic sense becomes refined, we see that physical sensations begin to evoke new patterns of thought. Whereas we may have reacted to the pain of a strained muscle with feelings of frustration, fear, and dependence on others for help, Kinetic Awareness gives us new ways to interpret the pain signals. We may still feel frustration, but we can also take it as a message to look at how we are treating ourselves and what the body is asking for. We can intercept potential problems while they are still only slight and readjust our way of using our body accordingly, towards what Maisel calls "positive conditions for health."[3] When the tension associated with pain releases, or when we are lucky enough to have no pain, the pleasurable physical feelings that result lead to a feeling of general happiness, which in itself is restorative. In fact, as Summers says, being able to enjoy our bodies for the pleasure of movement is one of the main goals of Kinetic Awareness. In describing her first Kinetic Awareness classes, Aileen Crow says, "I had immediate results. . . . I just fell in love with it. It was like an hour and a half of being entranced each week. And all those things I did in classes, I still use, all the time." As we are able to enjoy our everyday physical selves more, occasional aches and pains become less of a problem, and we can enjoy the good feelings of the body that we may have missed before becoming aware.

The slow pace of the work makes it possible for us to quiet our mind's usual chatter and begin to separate true feelings from memory of feelings or anticipation of feelings. Doing a task that is simple yet rich in potential discoveries, such as moving one part of the body very slowly and gently, we can gradually observe and feel more and more of ourselves. The body becomes interesting rather than confusing, overwhelming, or frightening. Both inward and outward awareness is sharpened so that, as several students I spoke with indicated, everything and every moment becomes a potential "teacher," a chance to be constantly aware.

Gindler described the interrelated nature, or connectedness, of life and of awareness work:

> There is a unity of experience—of one experience with another and all experience together—in which all the thousand-fold occurrences in life become inseparably connected. This unity must be so fully thought through and sensed through that it becomes an essential part of the person, by which he is led intuitively in every moment. Not that it is a possession which he has gradually acquired and can display on command, but rather something that is there for him immediately and without reflection in response to sudden stimulus.[4]

Yoga and Kinetic Awareness

Another practice which "becomes an essential part of the person," to use Gindler's words, is Yoga. Yoga is a much older, more spiritually oriented practice than any of the body therapies, but there are many interesting parallels between the two approaches to self-improvement. Since several people I spoke with compared bodywork with meditation, and as I am a practitioner of Yoga myself, I have included it in this discussion.

Yoga has its origins thousands of year ago in India as a way of life and a spiritual path. The goal of Yoga is to elevate everyday consciousness so that we can experience the profound joy and wisdom that is always inside but that we only rarely glimpse. Yoga offers the chance to clear away unwanted tensions, habits, and mental states in favor of openness, flexibility, and strength in both mind and body. What is actually done bears little resemblance to body therapies, but the general processes and many of the benefits are strikingly similar.

The practice of Yoga has many facets. The most common ones are meditation, called Dhyana Yoga in Sanskrit, and physical exercises, called Hatha Yoga. Meditation consists of sitting silently with a specific inward mental focus (different schools of Yoga follow different specific instructions) in order to calm the mind and experience our deeper selves. This process is often compared with watching the ripples of a pool subside. When the surface is clear, we can see the beauty of the reflected surroundings and of the depths below. Similarly, when we observe the bodymind calmly and without judgment or goals, extraneous tensions dissolve and we can enjoy both inward and outward awareness with more clarity and pleasure.

In Hatha Yoga, we assume physical postures that affect the body on four levels: 1) the muscles and joints are stretched and strengthened, 2) the internal digestive organs are toned, 3) the mind and emotions are calmed, and 4) spiritual awareness is enhanced. There are several hundred classical postures that have been specified to have certain benefits. Many of these are extremely difficult; it is clearly a lifelong undertaking.

Yoga requires a willingness to go slowly, to accept ourselves for what we are, and to witness the various things that happen as we progress. It is about being sensitive to the process, rather than striving to achieve anything "correct." There is an implicit recognition of inner resources, of an inward intelligence that we must get to know and be able to honor. While describing another bodywork technique, Anne-Reily defined a central part of Yoga: "A lot of it is doing away with the self-destructive devil that lives within all of us . . . the more you do it, the more aware you become. Like peeling away layer after layer of debris, and really finding more and more understanding, awareness, and inner knowledge. Not assumed knowledge but the innate knowledge."

Students have often described Kinetic Awareness as being very meditative, saying that they slip into a state of inner alertness that they would not have any other way. Pauline Oliveros underscored its similarities to meditation, saying, "The work has the appearance of being very simple, but it isn't. It's very dynamic and very complex and it takes a long time. It's gentle work, but it's very close to meditation, in that it's the accumulation day by day that has a very powerful effect."

There is a depth to the process of Yoga just as in Kinetic Awareness; effects are felt in all aspects of daily life—physical, mental, and emotional. As counterproductive tendencies begin to disappear, students feel more balanced, aware, responsible for their own state of health, and free to make choices about how to live their lives.

Kinetic Awareness—a foundation for growth

Although Kinetic Awareness shares many basic assumptions about the bodymind with other techniques, its specialty is helping us to bring our attention to the simplest components of body awareness and movement. "It's a foundation. . . ," Oliveros points out, "a preparation and security. . . . It can prepare you for any of the other types of movement disciplines."

After doing Kinetic Awareness for two years, Tom decided to try another bodymind technique, and he believes that he couldn't have done it without the skills he had gained with Kinetic Awareness. He had a different perspective on his bodymind, supported by the skill of moving slowly, the patience to listen to his body, and the confidence that easier movement was indeed possible for him.

Anne-Reily, who has also done other bodywork techniques, elaborates. "Some individuals would benefit from studying Kinetic Awareness before other techniques. Many people are not kinesthetically attuned to their bodies. They are unclear as to what their joints do, or exactly where they are located. They have mental pictures of their bodies but find once they begin moving that they have an inaccurate conception of where the movement is actually occurring." She added that the slow movement of the first phase of Kinetic Awareness is a revelation in itself, removing the censorship that often dulls our experience of our bodies. "When you have to move that slowly," she said, "you can't by-pass those little problem spots."

Many of the people I spoke with had this to say—that Kinetic Awareness is a prerequisite not just for other bodymind techniques, but also for activities such as sports, performing, or the martial arts. The skills and awareness gained are so basic that learning anything else becomes much easier and more rewarding. It's like having a chance to formulate our own map of the bodymind so that we have all our options open. With the understanding and coordination gained from Kinetic Awareness, we can pursue any type of exercise with more safety and confidence.

"To know is not enough"

Is there anyone who would not benefit from a study of Kinetic Awareness? It is possible that some people may feel too much anxiety about working slowly, about taking responsibility for their own body, or about what they might find out. In such a case, physical and mental defenses might be accentuated by the work. No one can do Kinetic Awareness for us; it is definitely a "do-it-yourself" method, requiring that the student be patient and willing to explore. Dancers and athletes may initially have to unlearn poor habits, but because of their commitment to body upkeep, they have strong motivation to continue doing the work once they begin to feel the benefits.

In my experience, Kinetic Awareness has been most meaningful to people who can suspend their own judgments of their body enough to accept the guidance of a good teacher, but then have the interest to maintain the process of growth in their own lives. As Gindler said, "To know is not enough. You must do it."[5] The teacher sets the example and provides suggestions for new experiences of awareness, but the students must make the technique their own.

Kinetic Awareness offers unique advantages within the general context of holistic systems. Three advantages are so important, that I would like to review them again:

1. There is no fixed sequence of instruction that a student must follow. The working process is adaptable in terms of choice of activity, intensity of the experience, and the results sought for.
2. The rubber balls function in many ways, as seen earlier, to allow easier, more direct discoveries and release of excess tension to occur.
3. Because movement with minimum effort is incorporated into the technique from the beginning, students learn to move all the parts of the body articulately, using any desired amount of tension. This skill is invaluable for anyone in any activity.

A natural way of living

All of the holistic systems could be accused of encouraging self-absorption and self-centeredness, leading to a society of narcissists. However, social changes start with people changing. As individuals become more self-aware and reponsible for their inward and outward experiences, social interaction and the culture at large will ultimately become more responsible and self-aware. As Dychtwald says in his book *Bodymind*:

> As I see it, the basic work has to be done at the starting point—on oneself. Social, cultural, and global interactions are dependent on the actions and movements of the individuals who make up the physical and psychological network of the group. For the group to change and improve itself, its members must first change and develop.[6]

Perhaps the bodymind therapies will soon become more widely accepted as a preventative approach, with educational programs for children to encourage healthy attitudes toward the body early in life and insurance coverage to acknowledge its place in the spectrum of health care.

Kinetic Awareness offers a vehicle for self-improvement; its benefits are many, and it is adaptable and appropriate for anyone who is interested in holistic approaches. The real core of this and any such method is the way we actually experience ourselves, through our senses and our understanding. As the mind and body work together, we find ways to come closer to a safe, natural way of living in our bodies—a way of living that enhances our sense of well-being from the inside out.

Notes

1. Alexander, *The Resurrection of the Body: The Essential Writings of F. Matthias Alexander,* page xxx.

2. Mary Alice Roche, in the Foreword to Charlotte Selver Foundation *Bulletin: Elsa Gindler 1885–1961,* vol. I, no. 10, page 3.

3. Alexander, *The Resurrection of the Body,* page xxx.

4. Gindler, "*Gymnastik* for Busy People," page 40.

5. Elsa Gindler, quoted in Elsa Henschke Durham in Charlotte Selver Foundation *Bulletin: Elsa Gindler 1885–1961,* vol. I, no. 10, page 40.

6. Dychtwald, *Bodymind,* page 261.

Where to Find a Teacher

The Kinetic Awareness Center is a nonprofit organization based in New York City. The center offers classes at various levels, special workshops, weekend intensives, and private sessions with certified teachers. A newsletter is published several times a year.

For more information about the center, please write:

Kinetic Awareness Center
P.O. Box 1050, Cooper Station
New York, N.Y. 10276

Annotated Bibliography

Books

Alexander, F. Matthias. *The Resurrection of the Body: The Essential Writings of F. Matthias Alexander.* Selected and introduced by Edward Maisel. Boston: Shambhala Publications, 1969.

A useful volume for studying bodymind theory from the words of one of its pioneers. Includes a long introduction by the editor summarizing Alexander's career.

Benjamin, Ben E., with Gale Borden. *Listen to Your Pain. The Active Person's Guide to Understanding, Identifying, and Treating Pain and Injury.* New York: Viking Press and Penguin Books, 1984.

A practical resource for interpreting pain signals in the body; anatomy, symptoms, and possible treatments for injuries are discussed in lay terms.

Bertherat, Therese, and Bernstein, Carol. *The Body Has Its Reasons.* New York: Random House, Pantheon Books, 1977.

Bertherat's story of discovering a bodymind integrative approach similar to Gindler's work, stressing self-awareness and honoring the wisdom of the body.

Brooks, Charles V. W. *Sensory Awareness. The Rediscovery of Experiencing.* New York: Viking Press, 1974.

Describes the attitude of awareness work and how our culture stresses thinking over sensing, with examples of bodymind experiments. Written by Charlotte Selver's husband and co-teacher.

Dowd, Irene. *Taking Root to Fly: Seven Articles in Functional Anatomy.* New York: Contact Collaborations, 1981.

Covers seven specific bodymind topics, with illustrations. Written by a prominent Ideokinesis teacher.

Dychtwald, Ken. *Bodymind.* New York: Harcourt Brace Jovanovich/Jove Publications, 1977.

A comprehensive account of the author's experience and research in psychosocial aspects of bodily behavior.

Feiss, George J. *Mind Therapies, Body Therapies: A Consumer's Guide.* Millbrae, California: Celestial Arts, 1979.

Concise descriptions of over 50 therapies, offering resource information for further study.

Feldenkrais, Moshe. *Awareness Through Movement.* New York: Harper and Row, 1972.

A thorough explanation of the author's theories in lay terms, and a description of basic lessons.

———. *Body and Mature Behavior: A Study of Anxiety, Sex, Gravitation, and Learning.* New York: International Universities Press, Inc., 1979.

A detailed and compelling book relating the topics in the subtitle to the development of human beings toward maturity.

Freud, Sigmund. *A General Selection from the Works of Sigmund Freud.* Edited by John Rickman. New York: Doubleday Anchor Books, 1957.

A useful anthology showing the general reader the progression of Freud's theories throughout his career.

Hill, Ann, ed. *A Visual Encyclopedia of Unconventional Medicine.* New York: Crown Publishers, 1979.

Illustrated articles on more than 100 approaches to bodymind health, from Oriental medicine to hypnosis. Resource information for further study.

Hulke, Malcolm, ed. *The Encyclopedia of Alternative Medicine and Self Help.* New York: Schocken Books, 1979.

A description of over 80 alternative health care techniques, with an extensive directory of resources.

Iyengar, B. K. S. *Light on Yoga.* New York: Schocken Books, 1979.

A basic modern text on Hatha Yoga. A long introduction explaining the philosophy of Yoga, followed by several hundred poses with instructions, a description of benefits, and photographs.

Johnson, Don. *The Protean Body*. New York: Harper Colophon Books, 1977.

A compelling discussion of the body as an energy system that is constantly in flux, expressing our life experiences and attitudes. Illustrated with case studies.

Kaslof, Leslie J. *Wholistic Dimensions in Healing. A Resource Guide*. New York: Doubleday, Dolphin Books, 1978.

A directory of over 60 holistic health care systems, with resource information for further study.

Kurtz, Ron, and Prestera, Hector. *The Body Reveals*. New York: Harper and Row, Quicksilver Books, 1976.

Presents a thorough system for diagnosis of personality through physical traits, with less emphasis on treatment, by a Rolfer and a Gestalt therapist.

Powell, J. Robin. "Body Awareness: The Kinetic Awareness Work of Elaine Summers." Ph.D. dissertation, New York University, 1985.

A thorough study of Kinetic Awareness theory and practice, tracing its antecedents and related fields of study.

Reich, Wilhelm. *Character Analysis*. New York: Farrar, Straus, and Giroux, 1972.

Reich's major work describing his bodymind theories, originally published in 1933.

———. *Selected Writings: An Introduction to Orgonomy*. New York: Harper and Row, 1976.

Excerpts from Reich's major books, with biographical information.

Schilder, Paul. *The Image and Appearance of the Human Body*. New York: International Universities Press, 1978.

A study of how we form a mental picture of our body and of the implications of body image on our behavior, written in the 1940s by a pioneer in psychiatry.

Speads, Carola H. *Ways to Better Breathing*. Great Neck, N.Y.: Felix Morrow, 1986.

An excellent, clearly written book guiding readers toward a better understanding of breathing, with practical suggestions.

Sweigard, Lulu E. *Human Movement Potential: Its Ideokinetic Facilitation*. New York: Harper and Row, 1974.

The author's method of neuromuscular reeducation, focusing on how postural alignment affects movement and how to facilitate improvements.

Todd, Mabel Elsworth. *The Thinking Body*. New York: Dance Horizons, 1968.

A detailed discussion of efficiency in posture and movement.

Articles and brochures

Bogen, J. E. "Some Educational Aspects of Hemisphere Specialization." *Dromenon* 506 (February 1979): 16–21.

Indications from brain research that nonverbal skills such as body awareness and movement will facilitate learning in other areas.

Cody, Kevin A., and Nelson, Arthur J., Jr. "The Effect of Verticality Perception on Body Balance in Normal Subjects." *Physical Therapy* 58 (January 1978): 16–41.

An interesting study of how people perceive their own body position in relation to external objects and how visual and kinesthetic cues are related.

Dowd, Irene. "Visualizing Movement Potential." *Dance Scope* 13 (Fall 1978): 24–35.

Principles and procedures of the Sweigard Ideokinesis method of neuromuscular reeducation.

Hatch, Frank W. "The Dancer as a Control System." *Psychological Perspectives on Dance,* Cord Dance Research Annual 11 (1978): 5–18.

A discussion of the physiological feedback a dancer uses to execute complex movements and how this feedback is interwoven with mental control.

Heaps, Richard. "Relating Physical and Psychological Fitness: A Psychological Point of View." *Journal of Sportsmedicine and Physical Fitness* 18 (December 1978): 399–408.

A study suggesting that comparative feedback about physical fitness will strongly affect a person's concept of his or her physicality.

Herskowitz, Morton. "The Body Therapies." *The Journal of Orgonomy* 13 (May 1979): 98–110.

An evaluation of several therapies based on or related to Reich's theories.

Houston, Jean. "Epilogue: Consider the Stradivarius." *Dromenon* 1 (February 1979): 40–42.

Presents the case for multiperceptual education, with more sensory experiences to enrich the learning process and encourage children to use different parts of their brains than are currently called upon by conventional education.

Hunt, Valerie. "The Biological Organization of Man to Move." *Impulse* (1968): 51–63.

From a lecture-demonstration discussing physiological principles of body movements, aspects of movement study, and body image.

Myers, Martha. "Body Therapies and the Modern Dancer: The New 'Science' in Dance Training." *Dance Magazine* (February 1980): 90–92.

Introducing her series on body therapies, Myers discusses the body-mind interplay and its role in dance training.

———. "Body Therapies and the Modern Dancer: Dance Training's New Frontier." *Dance Magazine* (July 1980): 78–82.

The conclusion of Myers' series on body therapies for dancers, discussing touch, body image, movement learning, and alignment.

Pew, Thomas W., Jr. "Biofeedback Seeks New Uses for Concept of Yoga." *Smithsonian* (December 1979): 106–14.

A description of uses for biofeedback in pain control, stressing bodymind interconnections.

Selver, Charlotte. "Sensory Awareness and Total Functioning." *General Semantics* Bulletin nos. 20 and 21 (1957).

———. "On Breathing." Caldwell, N. J.: Charlotte Selver Foundation, n.d.

Selver, Charlotte, and Brooks, Charles V. W. "Report on Work in Sensory Awareness and Total Functioning." Springfield, Ill.: *Explorations in Human Potentialities,* 1966.

Explanations of the theories and practices involved with Selver's Sensory Awareness work.

Sensory Awareness Foundation (formerly Charlotte Selver Foundation). *Sensory Awareness: The Work of Selver.* Caldwell, N.J.: 1973.

———. *Bulletin: Elsa Gindler 1885–1961*, vol. I, no. 10 (Summer 1978).

———. *Bulletin: Elsa Gindler 1885–1961*, vol. II, no. 10 (Winter 1981).

———. *Bulletin: Elsa Gindler 1885–1961*, no. 11 (Winter 1983).

Documenting the work of Gindler and those who followed her, these publications provide a valuable written resource on awareness work.

Speads, Carola H. "Physical Re-Education: What It Is and What It Is Not." *Somatics,* vol. 1, no. 2 (Spring 1977): 21–23.

An eloquent statement on why people need awareness work, how it relates to other methods, and what can be gained from its use.

———. "Somatics Interview with Carola Speads." *Somatics,* vol. 3, no. 2 (Spring/Summer 1981): 10–13.

Interesting historical account of Speads' work with Gindler.

Wooster, Ann-Sargent. "Elaine Summers: Moving To Dance." *The Drama Review*, vol. 24, no. 4 (December 1980): 59–70.

Chronicles Summers' development of Kinetic Awareness and how she uses the work as an underlying structure for choreography.

Kinetic Awareness:
Discovering Your Bodymind
was designed by Romeo Enriquez,
typeset by Ira Ungar, and produced by the
Publishing Center for Cultural Resources.
The Publishing Center is a nonprofit organization
founded in 1973 to help nonprofit educational
institutions and associations become
effective publishers. Its services, which
now extend to over 150 organizations
throughout the United States, are made
possible by grants from public agencies and
private foundations and corporate contributions.
The Publishing Center is located in New York City.